Heal Environmental Illness
and
Reclaim Your Life!

Learn new techniques to clear
allergies and sensitivities
and rebuild your life.

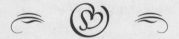

—*A message of hope from*
Lorraine Smith

Diveena ♡ Publications
Chelmsford, MA

Diveena Publications, Chelmsford, MA 01824
© 2000 by Diveena ♡ Publications
All rights reserved.

HEAL ENVIRONMENTAL ILLNESS
AND
RECLAIM YOUR LIFE!

For information,
Address: Diveena Publications,
            PO Box 413, Chelmsford, MA 01824
Fax: 978-250-1938
Email: LSmithDCH@aol.com

First edition published 2000.

Cover Artwork by William Ho
Cover Design by Debbie de Haas
Printed by *BookMasters,* Mansfield, OH

ISBN (paperback): 0–9675624–0–6
Library of Congress Card Catalog Number:
99–96135

This book is printed with 100 percent soy ink on
natural paper in the United States of America.

Dedications

To David

I *would like to dedicate this book to my wonderful and brave husband, David. You protected me physically and emotionally during the endless days of suffering. You stood by my side and believed in me. You gave me the courage to find the answer, and you never wavered in your love for me.*

To Mother

I *would also like to dedicate this work to my mother, whose constant love and caring gave me the strength to carry on. You believed in me and prayed for me. You kept me alive that very terrible summer, and that, I will never forget.*

To Robert and Patricia

I *would like to thank Dr. Robert Sampson and Patricia Hughes, my healers, my friends. You took my hand and led me out of the pain and suffering in which I was living. You taught me new ideas and gave me a new belief in myself. You shared your gift of healing, and helped me to save my life.*

A Poem of Hope

Your smile is weak,
Your eyes are dry.
You cry inside . . .
And I know why.

Your life seems ruined,
The joy is gone.
It's hard each day
To carry on,

but

There will be a rainbow
And there will be a light,
And a ray of dear hope
That life can be right.

Dreams will reopen,
As joy reappears.
Your smile will strengthen,
As your eyes shed their tears.

The deep pain will empty
And life will be sweet.
Just like a kitten . . .
You'll land on your feet!

—Lorraine Smith

CONTENTS

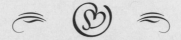

Contents   7

FOREWORD

When I agreed to review Dr. Smith's book, I thought it would be a boring task. The book came sooner than expected, and after taking one look at this thick manuscript, I just left it on the coffee table, not wanting to even begin. However, I had agreed to do this, so I reluctantly went on to the "task."

I tell you, I almost couldn't put this book down!

I congratulate the people who stood by her and helped Lorri recover her health. I also hold in admiration her husband, whose loyalty and love must be tremendous.

I hold in contempt those people who laughed at her and insisted that she was not ill. Were they blind? Do they have no compassion? Should people like these be allowed to work in the helping professions?

I have never read a book that shows so much bravery and sincerity. Dr. Smith shows in her book a vast knowledge of alternative therapies. She also shows what the mind can do with proper training and how much you can accomplish when you believe in yourself. This is a book everyone should read to gain inspiration and encouragement.

I would say, "God bless you," but He already has, and I know you are passing those blessings on.

—A. M. Krasner, Ph.D.
Founder and CEO
American Institute of Hypnotherapy

PREFACE

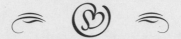

I had waited to see this particular doctor for the month since my injury. Now as I walked to my car, I felt numb. He had given my condition a name. It was *Multiple Chemical Sensitivity* (MCS) or *Environmental Illness* (EI). These words meant nothing to me. I had never heard of either condition. But what I kept hearing in my ears were his final comments. "There is no cure. You will have to find your own cure."

As I got into my car I wondered how this had happened to me: Two months ago I had been fine, and very happy. Now my life seemed to be in ruins. I could hardly function. I had waited for this medical expert to help me and now he only turned me away with a doubtful shake of his head. He said that there is little understanding about this condition. Some doctors don't even believe in it.

If they don't understand it, how was I supposed to? What does it mean to be sensitive to chemicals? What chemicals? How does this happen? I was totally confused.

I can only say now, that if I had known that day what I would go through, I do not know how I would have found the courage to drive home and begin the ordeal.

DISCLAIMER

*T*his book deals with a condition known as Environmental Illness (EI), also called Multiple Chemical Sensitivity (MCS). I will use these terms interchangeably throughout the text. This illness is characterized by multiple allergies and sensitivities to substances in the environment, including molds, dusts, foods, and especially chemicals. Very minute exposures to these substances may result in serious reactions of various types. Many organs can be involved.

This book is not a substitute for traditional medical care. If a health problem arises, the services of a competent medical professional should be sought.

This work merely provides suggestions for new and effective treatments from which many people have been benefiting. Not all treatments work for all people! *You* are the ultimate judge of what is appropriate for your own successful healing. If any technique does not resonate with you, or if it may cause any discomfort, discontinue it immediately. Always be selective and cautious—your body is very special and your individual needs should be respected.

Some of the names herein have been altered to provide anonymity. The fictitious names are as follows: Dr. English, Dr. Green, Dr. Kane, Dr. Peterson, Dr. Wyner, Attorney Sands, and my personal friends. All other names are actual, so that you may contact some of the excellent physicians and healers, if you so desire. Their addresses are listed in an appendix at the conclusion of this work.

The purpose of this book is to educate and enlighten. Diveena Publications and the author shall assume neither liability nor responsibility should problems occur or be alleged to occur as a direct or indirect result of reading this book.

If you do not wish to be bound by the above, you may return this book, accompanied by a sales receipt, to the publisher, and your money will be refunded.

ACKNOWLEDGMENTS

I wish to extend my sincerest gratitude to Erika Hetzner, the editor of this book. On a technical level, she carefully corrected and adjusted grammar and punctuation. However, it was on a deeper level that she brought life to my story. From the beginning, she believed in my message and recognized that this book could deliver hope and love to so many people suffering with Environmental Illness.

Gently, she encouraged me to invite you, the reader, into my world to experience personally the challenges of living with EI. She sought for my heartfelt honesty and my clear intentions. Initially, expressing my true feelings was difficult, for they were so painful. It was Erika who allowed me to feel safe doing so. Therefore, if you feel anger at the doctors who insulted me, sorrow at my many disappointments, and joy at my smallest improvements, it was Erika who delicately directed me to lovingly escort you through these adventures.

My gratitude is also extended to William Ho, the fine artist who created the cover artwork and illustrations for my book. How talented and gifted a young man he is! I wish him a wonderful, fulfilling, and bright future!

I would like to express my appreciation to Debbie de Haas, the very talented designer of the book's cover. She understood the level of care and concern I held for this project. Cheerfully, she joined in to produce a cover in perfect harmony with this book.

INTRODUCTION

*T*his is a true story! The pages set before you are those of my journey through the most difficult and challenging years of my life! When I was stricken with Environmental Illness, everything as I knew it ended. To continue on meant total changes and alterations in every aspect of my existence. Nothing seemed to work any more! The message from the allopathic medical community was consistent—"no cure, no cure." There seemed to be no way out! To live was unbearable; to die was unthinkable!

With my loving husband, David, by my side, we faltered along until the life-saving answers arrived—wonderful, enlightening revelations, that I now share with you to use as you see fit. My message is not one of anger and resentment, but rather one of hope and determination. By reaching deep within yourself, you may discover the power to heal and go on to reclaim your life!

PART I

On my journey of life, a roadblock is set before me. I cannot proceed. I must evaluate and consider an alternate route, for none is presented to me. I cannot do this alone. I will ask for God's help to find my way around the obstacle.

Chapter 1

I AM INJURED

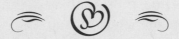

*I*t was September of 1994—time to return to school. This would mark my twentieth year as a teacher. I had taught many subjects in my career. They included humanities, social studies, French, Spanish, German, and now American history. I had been assigned to the eighth-grade level the previous year, and had really enjoyed it. Now I was very pleased to be assigned to that level again. I could add to my program and make it even better. I was excited to see my friends as well. Teaching was my lifelong career and I loved it!

The faculty had received a notice during the summer that the school roof was being replaced. I didn't know what this entailed, but had wondered if the work would be completed by September.

As I entered the auditorium, I spotted two of my best friends, Jenny and Pat. They beckoned to me to sit down between them.

We were all giggly and excited. It never ceased to amaze me how, after all these years, I continued to have little butterflies in my stomach on this first day back. There was such a feeling of anticipation. So much would be new, including the children and my team of teachers.

The three of us sat listening to the superintendent make his usual opening address. Once in a while we glanced at one another and smiled. We were like schoolgirls—all excited and a little apprehensive.

While we listened to the opening speeches, the hammering and pounding was evident on the roof. The superintendent announced that the roof replacement had not gone well over the summer and had to continue during the fall. He was sorry about the noise. If only noise was all I would contend with!

After the speeches, it was time to return to our classrooms and prepare for the next day. Pat, Jenny, and I said good-bye. They were on their way to the other middle school, where they taught. It had been a pleasant morning.

My room was very large, with a high ceiling. This was the room I had been assigned to last year. It felt very comfortable. My desk seemed to welcome me, and I looked around at all the familiar smaller desks and bookcases. It was so nice to be back.

Since my room was an inside room, the windows were at the top of the side walls overlooking the lower roof of the outer perimeter of the school. The custodian had to open and close these windows for me from the outside, by standing on the lower roof.

This day, the windows were open, but a foul odor drifted in. As I worked about the room, I couldn't seem to escape it. The smell actually seemed to change as the morning wore on. At first, it smelled like glue. Then it resembled nail polish or acetone. After a couple more hours, a very heavy rubber-glue smell filled the room.

Most of my attention was focused on the preparation for the children's first day of school; however, the smell kept distracting me. I wondered what it was, but I assured myself that it must be safe. Certainly, the administration wouldn't let us breathe anything dangerous!

The next day was Wednesday, the first official day of school when the children would be present and I would be extremely busy. I was to teach six classes a day with each class remaining in my room for about forty-five minutes. That day, as each group entered my classroom, they inquired about the smell. The workers were directly above us on the roof. I could see them working when I looked out the high window that faced the other roof level. The strong odor was ever present, but I was too busy then to inquire about the smell. I thought that the administration must surely have made certain that the substances were safe for children and teachers.

Friday, two days later, I was beginning to feel weak. At one point, when I had kept my classroom door closed for the entire period, fumes collected in my room. I felt as if I would pass out. After making it through that class, I opened the door to the hallway where the air seemed to be better. The next period was a preparation period for me, which didn't involve having students in my room. I left for the front office, where there was air conditioning and where I regained my strength. I was getting concerned about the fumes in my classroom. I didn't know what they were and I wondered whether or not they were safe to breathe. Why hadn't anyone acknowledged the fumes or their effects? I had begun to feel frustrated and annoyed. So much work was required this opening week of school. It was a tense and very tiring time. There wasn't a free moment. Was it my responsibility to monitor the substances used in the roof repair as well?

Over the weekend, I gradually recovered. I felt much better by Sunday and prepared to return to work for the following week. Little did I know that it would be a week that would change the rest of my life!

I felt fairly well Monday, but by Tuesday I began to feel seriously ill. It was a sultry, hot, humid day. There seemed to be no fresh air to breathe. Within minutes of entering my classroom, students were becoming ill. Some became extremely dizzy; others began having what appeared to be asthma attacks. I sent the affected students to the nurse. Finally, by fifth period, the fumes were very heavy and they were affecting me as well. I became very faint and could barely muster enough strength to assist my students. I knew that I needed to keep my mind focused to help them, but I felt as if I were looking through a haze. I could hardly function. Struggling to keep myself alert, I did manage to get the students outside. We had to move far away from the building because the air surrounding the school gave off a terrible odor. The entire class and I were lying on the ground. I could not understand why we were so ill. What could we be breathing?

When the closing bell rang, the children walked over to their buses; some with headaches, some dizzy, and some clutching their inhalers. What a way to return home!

My body felt exhausted and weak. My head throbbed on the right side. I was nauseous, and my face and sinuses were burning. It was difficult to breathe; all I could do when I arrived home was lie down for the rest of the afternoon and evening.

The next day, Wednesday, I still felt ill and so did the children. We hadn't recovered from the fumes of the day before. My head continued to ache, and all the other symptoms persisted. I was still shaky and weak. The children expressed their dismay over their reactions to the fumes. They looked tired and ill. They complained of headaches and asthma attacks that had lasted all night.

That day I decided not to teach in my classroom. I promised my students that they would not have to endure another day like the day before. They were relieved. Instead, for the day, we went to the library where the air was clear. We all felt somewhat better that day. I intended to use the library again the next day; however, that Thursday, the first period class entered the library and then the children informed me that the fumes were there as well. The workers were overhead. Now I didn't know what to do or where to go. We needed fresh air and we couldn't find any. Finally, I decided to speak to the principal. I told him that the children and I were sick from the fumes. When I asked him what we were breathing, he said they were adhesives and solvents. This didn't mean anything to me. I didn't know much about chemicals and I wasn't given any names of the products.

The principal seemed exasperated. He said he had to finish the roof. What could he do?

With an aching head, I looked directly at him and stated emphatically, "This building isn't safe for these children. The day before, a classroom full of students was outside, lying on the ground. Shouldn't something be done?"

Again he held his position. "The roof has to be finished. I can't close the whole building."

"Perhaps we could use the other middle school and have double sessions until the construction is complete and the air is clear. We have done this before when this school was being built," I reminded him.

He dismissed this idea. "It would be too inconvenient."

There was nothing I could say to convince him that the school wasn't healthy for children and teachers. My fatigue and headache were taking over and after the talk, we decided that I should stay home until the roof was finished, as I had accumulated over one hundred sick days. He thought that the roof should be finished by the next week anyway. But what about the children?

He said he would take care of things.

I remained at home for the following two weeks. My body felt extremely weak. I could hardly summon enough strength to get up in the morning. I ached all over. Each night I awoke struggling to breathe. My head throbbed on the right side constantly. I had no idea what was happening. I just knew that something was not right.

I attempted to call the owner of the roofing company to inquire about what chemicals we were breathing and how long their effects would last. I also needed to know if they would be continuing to use them. Finally, I reached him. He said that they would be using the solvents every day until the roof was finished. Then he said that I should not worry because they were, "nothing more than white glue!"

I did not have a vast knowledge of chemicals, but even I knew this was absurd. I had used white glue for many years in classroom projects, and I had never felt like this before! Still, I could not get any accurate answers as to what I was breathing. The owner had just tried to placate me instead of giving me any facts. I needed to know what the fumes were that were hurting me. Nobody seemed to take this issue seriously, and I was getting frustrated.

I then called OSHA (Occupational Safety and Health Agency). Much to my surprise, the person I spoke with informed me that they only had jurisdiction over the private sector. They had no say in the schools. I was told to call the Massachusetts Department of Education. I did so and found out that they, too, had no regulations or safety codes for air quality in the schools. This amazed me. Who, then, cared what happened to us in the schools? I tried calling the Division of Occupational Hygiene. A man I spoke with showed some concern. He said that any time a rubber roof is applied, there are many complaints. He said the odor is terrible. When I inquired about the safety of the children, he was kind, but had no intention of checking the situation.

I was so disappointed. I saw now that there were no controls governing air quality in Massachusetts public schools, thus teachers and children were very vulnerable. I could not find a single agency to help. I kept thinking of the children breathing those fumes and I felt sad for them. There seemed to be nothing I could do to help them.

It had been two weeks since I had left. I had begun to feel a bit stronger. I drove by the school to see if the roof had been finished. The workers were still there. I called one over and asked if they were through applying the adhesives. He said that they would not be using them the next day due to the predicted rain.

I had much to do and I had missed my students. I planned to go back to school that next day. This turned out to be a very big mistake.

I was very nervous that night. I slept very little. I was still feeling ill, but I needed and wanted to get back to my students. I hadn't even had the opportunity to begin the school year or to get to know them.

The next day, Thursday, was bright and sunny and, much to my dismay, the roofers were using buckets and buckets of adhesives over my roof. I became increasingly dizzy and ill. This time it was unbearable. The nausea was horrible and my head was pounding. My face and sinuses burned. I felt terrible. I just barely made it through the day. Upon my return home, I retired to bed.

My husband, David, helped me prepare supper that night. He was getting very concerned. As we sat at the table, he began asking me some questions. "What is happening at school?"

I replied, "I am breathing 'adhesives and solvents.'"

Being trained in the field of science, he inquired, "Which ones exactly?"

I said, "I don't know. I was only told they were 'adhesives and solvents.'"

He looked very serious. He had been worrying about me since the first week of school. Now my health seemed to be rapidly declining. He firmly insisted, "You must find out exactly what you are breathing. You know you are not supposed to inhale adhesives and solvents—and certainly not all day long, every day!" David was very intelligent and usually very calm, but this evening he seemed exasperated about the situation in the school. His next comment touched me deeply, "And what about all those young children? Is anybody concerned about what those adhesives and solvents are doing to them?"

Very wearily, I explained about my conversation with the principal. There seemed to be no real concern about the children, just the completion of the roof! Due to the heavy nausea and throbbing headache, I couldn't seem to eat much. After supper, I began walking back to the bedroom. David accompanied me and sat in the chair beside our bed. I promised him I would request specific information about the chemicals I was breathing. As I rested my aching head against the pillow, I said, "Don't worry, David, the roof is almost finished. Maybe I can stick it out."

I slept only a few hours because I felt so ill, but the next day I dragged myself to work. I had no other room to go to during the first several hours of the day. However, I arranged to use a friend's classroom on the other side of the building during the afternoon hours. His room had no fumes and I thought that maybe I would be safe for a couple of hours anyway. Unfortunately, I couldn't make it through the day. My body couldn't take any more. I could barely stand up and I was unable to think clearly. I was having breathing problems and I was extremely nauseous. My skin and sinuses were constantly burning. I spoke to the principal who said I should leave. He was understanding, and yet when I inquired about the children left to breathe these fumes, he only said that he had to finish the roof. The nurse just simply sent the sick children home each day.

I arrived home that Friday extremely ill. I couldn't seem to think clearly. My head ached on the right side. I was nauseated and struggling to breathe. My sinuses were completely burned and blocked. I went to bed to rest. When my husband arrived home, I was lying down, something I seemed to being doing a lot lately. He prepared dinner and I tried to eat. It was then that something happened to me that I shall never forget. I felt this searing, gut-wrenching pain going through my body on my right side. My whole insides felt like they were being ripped apart. It felt like it involved every fiber of my being. I bent over and held my side. I didn't move for a long time. Finally the pain subsided. I knew that something had gone terribly wrong deep within my body.

Chapter 2

THE INJURY CHANGES MY LIFE

During that fall, I spent October and November attempting to find some answers to help me resolve my perplexing health problems. The more I searched, the more frightened I became. The medical community seemed as puzzled as I about this mysterious condition.

Saturday, the day after my discussion with David, we went to my internist. I was very ill and Dr. Reid confirmed that my condition was a result of my exposure to the solvents and adhesives. He advised me not to return to the school until the roof was entirely finished or until the air was much colder and it ceased to outgas. The doctor explained that the fumes would be stronger when the weather was hot because the solvents evaporate into the air. I couldn't understand much of what he said that day because my head throbbed and I was very confused. Words were just mumbled and blurry to me. Something was wrong with my head.

That next week, I was bedridden. Finally, one night, David suggested that we take a ride to get me out of the house. I got up, got dressed, and got into his relatively new Jeep. As we began to ride, I became very ill. I struggled to breathe, my faced burned, and my head ached even more. I became dizzy. What was happening to me? We drove home. This situation was very bizarre. We had been using this vehicle all summer with absolutely no difficulty. Now, it made me feel terrible. What could the explanation be?

Later that week, we tried again, only we used my car. This time I was fine in the car. We drove to a store to look at some objects my husband needed. We had always wandered through this store together before. But this time, after ten minutes, I almost passed out. The room went dark, my head ached, and my face burned. We had to go home. Now I was very frightened.

Upon my return, I fell into bed, exhausted, and very worried. David just sat beside me to make sure I was all right. Was I all right? What in the world was happening to me? My body felt horrible and I had no idea why!

Later, when I attempted to accomplish other "simple" tasks such as reading, watching television, or using my computer, I would become ill. My already distressing symptoms were becoming accentuated. The right side of my head began to hurt all the time, but it would pound unbearably when I tried to look at my computer screen. My face would burn and I couldn't breathe when I watched television or when I read a book. Now I was baffled and very worried. I had never experienced anything like this before. Surely it would go away soon! I couldn't imagine living like this.

I called my internist and told him of the latest developments. He seemed to have an idea about what was going on. He recommended a specialist in environmental medicine. I made an appointment and waited to see Dr. Peterson.

Meanwhile, I heard that another teacher from our school was rushed to the hospital by ambulance. He had had a severe asthma attack. Now I knew that the fumes I had been inhaling were very hazardous. Mr. Insogna, from the Division of Occupational Hygiene, called my house and asked how I was doing. Since another teacher was having difficulty, his agency was getting concerned. Mr. Insogna promised that he would find out exactly what we were breathing and notify me when he received the information.

It took him a week to obtain the Material Safety Data Sheets (MSDS). These are sheets prepared by the manufacturer of the chemicals that explain the proper usage of the chemicals and their possible side effects. They list precautions and explanations.

Mr. Insogna called, informing me that I had been exposed to very dangerous chemicals and should see a doctor. I explained that I had already seen a doctor and was waiting to see another. Mr. Insogna wished me good luck and said that he would send me the MSDS sheets he had just received.

When I received the sheets, I read over the information they contained. The chemicals included toluene, xylene, heptane, acetone, aliphatic petroleum distillates, ammonium montmorillonite, naphtha, isopropyl alcohol, and so on. There were several sheets with lists of toxic chemicals all containing warnings against inhaling these fumes. Some of the effects of chronic exposure include:

> irritation of skin, eyes, and mucous membranes of upper respiratory tract on prolonged repeated contact, dermatitis and defatting of the skin. Prolonged

overexposure to solvents have been associated with permanent brain and nervous system damage.[1]

Other sheets went on to say:

Chronic exposure may cause reversible liver and kidney injury. Overexposure may result in headache, dizziness, fatigue, nausea, loss of consciousness, and even asphyxiation. Reports have associated repeated and prolonged occupational overexposure to toluene with high frequency hearing loss based on animal tests.[2]

These were not harmless chemicals! I wondered what constituted overexposure. Was there a limited exposure time before someone was considered injured? What was the tolerance level for children? There was nothing about these issues on the sheets. I knew I had reached that time limit, for I was very ill. I couldn't understand why we had not been informed that we would be breathing these toxic and dangerous substances. Why was the school left open while this kind of renovation was going on? The MSDS sheets indicated that the vapors of these chemicals were significantly heavier (2–4 times) than air. Many of the ceiling tiles had been removed because they had been ruined by the leaking roof. These openings allowed the fumes to easily sink into the building. Didn't the principal even investigate what we would be breathing? Especially the chil-

---

[1] **Chapter 2:** Material Safety Data Sheets, Elastomeric Sealant, Synthetic Rubber/Resin mastic, Rubber-based Sealant, Butyl Adhesive (Carlisle, PA: Carlisle Syntec Inc.)
[2] Ibid.

dren? I will never understand why this happened, but I realized that all of my energy must be focused on recovery and not wasted on anger or regret.

During the time I waited for my appointment with the environmental specialist, the principal submitted my worker's compensation claims. He had to do this for the other teacher as well. I called my union president to inform her about my injury. I was surprised and disappointed to receive a very polite refusal to assist me in any way. The union, I was informed, only helped members who were accused of a wrongdoing. If a member got hurt, he was on his own! I had paid union dues for twenty years and now I needed help. They just turned away. I needed advice about what I should do. None was given.

I continued to have more and more problems with everyday substances. I couldn't breathe after I cleaned my bathroom or washed the dishes. I had always used the same soaps, and yet now they made me sick. I was confused. How long would this last? Should I just wait it out? I was very weak and tired. My head ached constantly on the right side. I was on asthma medicine to breathe. My sinuses were hurting me and I could not breathe through them. Still more and more tasks became impossible. I found that I could not be in a store at all without serious symptoms. What was this all about?

I avoided reading for more than ten minutes, using my computer, and watching television. Each of these activities provoked reactions. It was a struggle—getting through each day without too many reactions, and trying to figure out what was happening. Nothing made sense. These were simple everyday activities. Why could I no longer perform them? My appointment with Dr. Peterson would be soon, and hopefully he could bring clarity to this situation. He would give me the answers I needed to help me recover. Most of my attention was spent trying to remain calm until I saw him.

By the time I had my appointment with Dr. Peterson, I had found a book, *Staying Well in a Toxic World,* by Lynn Lawson, which I was attempting to read. It contained a definition of the condition called Multiple Chemical Sensitivity, which read " . . . illness reactions associated with exposure to more than one chemical, at significantly lower exposure levels than would cause noticeable illness in the general population . . . [3]

This seemed to describe exactly what I was experiencing. I showed the book to the doctor and asked if this was what was happening to me. He laughed and said it was, but that I should throw the book away and ignore the precautions about avoiding chemicals. "Keep living and going out." He said, "Don't isolate yourself. It isn't healthy."

I was pleased to hear that. I loved going out and being with other people. He continued, "Indeed you do have Multiple Chemical Sensitivity (MCS), also called Environmental Illness (EI)."

I felt worried, and inquired, "How can I get better so that I can return to work?"

He replied quickly, "You can go back to work part time in December. However . . . there is no cure." He continued, "You will just have to find your own cure."

I was baffled. "How am I supposed to go back to work if I can not even read a book, use a computer, or even watch a television?"

---

[3] Lynn Lawson, *Staying Well in a Toxic World* (Chicago, IL: The Noble Press, Inc. 1993), 34.

Dr. Peterson merely added, "Just go back to work and see how you feel."

He didn't address the issue of my existing sensitivities and basically wanted me to ignore them. Sure, I would be happy to go back to work, but I was also intelligent and knew that I would have to heal myself first. Dr. Peterson left me so confused and he was one of the experts! He said first that he would submit a form to worker's compensation, and then he said that he represented them. It wasn't clear to me at the time, but later I began to realize that I also had to deal with the game of worker's comp wanting me to work no matter how sick I was. This was all new to me and I didn't understand. The doctor had done his duty for the insurance company and had recommended that I go back to work. Now I was supposed to find my own cure!

That next week, during the beginning of November, I tried to carry on as he advised. I went into stores and used my usual soaps and cleaners. I tried to ignore the problem and not isolate myself. Within days, my health had deteriorated. I could no longer get out of bed. Hadn't I done what the doctor ordered? I called his office and spoke to his nurse. I related the turn of events. The next day, the doctor called. He told me to come back in to see him. I informed him that I was too ill to go anywhere, but when I recovered enough to get out of bed, I would indeed come in to see him. Three weeks later, I was in his office. He listened as I recounted the results of following his advice. I told him I was trying not to isolate myself, but that it didn't seem to be working. He was confused and admitted that he didn't really understand my illness. He said that I should go to someone else. He gave no specific recommendation. Again, he advised, "You have to find your own cure."

As my appointment ended, he asked, "Whose doctor am I?" I was baffled by his very strange question. I replied that he was my doctor of course. He knew I didn't comprehend what he meant so he rephrased the question. "No, I mean, who is paying me?" I understood a little more. I guessed he meant, was I paying him or was the insurance company for worker's compensation paying him. Realizing that he was concerned about being paid, I assured him that I had selected him and needed him to help me. I would pay him myself. Then he handed me a slip as I left. It read "totally disabled."

I walked away from his office in a daze. I didn't go to him to be diagnosed as *totally disabled.* I had gone to him for help. Did the diagnosis change because I was paying him? Last time he said that I could go back to work. This time I was totally disabled! He admits that he has no idea about my condition. He is the expert! What was I going to do to get well?

As I walked to the parking lot, I felt numb. Nothing was making any sense. My life was falling apart and there were no answers. My heart was pounding and my body felt weak. Sitting in the front seat of my car, I just stared out the window. If this so-called expert had no idea about Multiple Chemical Sensitivity, what was I going to do about recovering from it? At that moment, I realized the magnitude of the situation I was in. Something was wrong with me and no one knew what it was. My hands shook and I started my car. Dr. Peterson's words kept repeating in my head, "There is no cure. You will have to find your own cure . . . your own cure."

This was the beginning of a quest that would take me on a year and a half journey. I did not ever return to teaching. It was soon apparent that I was dealing with a very serious situation and needed to find some answers. The symptoms simply would not go away, and I was totally confused.

Now I was on my own. Nobody was helping me. The two doctors had no clear explanation. What does it mean for me to be chemically sensitive? I wondered: which chemicals are the problem? Should I avoid some or all of them? . . . I had so many questions and no answers. I couldn't figure out why I had reacted to my easy chair when I sat down. Were there "chemicals" in my chair? I had never considered that before. I now had reactions in every room of my home. I didn't know where the chemicals were that were affecting me. This whole problem was a mystery to me and I kept getting sicker and sicker.

I was becoming very depressed. Every morning I cried in my pillow when my husband left for work—I missed my classroom and the children. All my adult years I had been a teacher. It was my identity, my life. It felt so unnatural to remain sick in bed with no purpose. Each day I was left alone to attempt to find some answers. My health was failing, and yet I kept thinking and hoping that this illness would just go away. It felt like I was living in a bad dream, and at any moment, I would wake up and the misery would be over.

Meanwhile, each day dragged by and I struggled on. My reactions continued relentlessly. I had a constant pain in my head on the right side. My neck and back had started to ache shortly after the exposure and they were still bothering me. I couldn't breathe out of my nose because my sinuses were still completely blocked. I generally felt exhausted and ill. My routine was very limited. Mostly I sat on the couch in my den upstairs by an open window. I had to have a window constantly open, because I couldn't seem to breathe if the window were shut. I had no idea why.

I could not read or watch TV. When I attempted to do these things, my face would burn and I couldn't breathe. I just sat alone in a kind of fog and wondered how this had happened to me.

Luckily, my dentist had heard about my plight and informed his very lovely wife, Glenda. She called me within minutes of hearing about my problem. She consoled me and shared her own experience of attempting to heal for many years. She told me about others who were also struggling with chronic illnesses. I called one woman who informed me about a support group for MCS in Massachusetts. After speaking with the leader, I felt hopeful about meeting others with the same condition. I prepared to attend a meeting one Monday night.

When I called for directions that afternoon, I spoke to the leader from the next state who was hosting the meeting. He asked if I had a "handicapped plate." I was stunned. I asked why I would have that. He said other members had them because they were handicapped. He also said that members wore masks and talked all evening about the trials of living with MCS. When I inquired whether they discussed ways to heal, he seemed surprised. He replied that there was no cure and that most of the members had been ill for a very long time.

Once again, I was hearing that same bleak message, "no cure, no cure." Was this true? Was there indeed "no cure?" Did a person who was chemically injured have to remain that way for the rest of his/her life? How could I bear this?

I hung up the phone. I felt frightened. I wasn't sure that I could handle seeing people in masks and wearing the other gear they might need. I couldn't seem to accept the illness as a permanent condition. I just could not go to a meeting and focus on the sadness of this illness all night. I wanted to focus on how to heal. There had to be a way! Indeed, I did need help with how to live and how to make accommodations for my altered life, but this wasn't the way I wanted to go about it. I knew that if I met with these people and talked constantly about MCS, I might never get well. It reminded me of a quote from Norman Cousin's book, *Anatomy of an Illness:*

> People have asked me what I thought when I was told by the specialists that my disease was progressive and incurable. The answer is simple. Since I didn't accept the verdict, I wasn't trapped in the cycle of fear, depression, and panic that frequently accompanies a supposedly incurable illness.[4]

I decided not to attend the meeting that night. I knew then that I had to direct my focus on healing and on believing that I could completely get well. I simply wouldn't accept the verdict that this was permanent and incurable. Instead, I made friends with some of the group members who were determined to heal, and I limited my exposure to others who had defeated attitudes—who had resigned themselves to this label of MCS forever. I had no answers for a cure, but I couldn't give in. I couldn't bear the thought of living, or rather *not living* for the rest of my life.

Slowly, a whole new group of people opened up to me. Through my phone network, I began to meet many wonderful people who were seriously injured chemically. Many of these people were educated professionals. They were kind and caring. Most of my new friends were women, and it seemed to us that the

---

[4] Norman Cousins, *Anatomy of an Illness* (New York, NY: Bantam Books, 1981), 45.

majority of MCS sufferers were indeed women. We did not know why this was so.

Each person I spoke with related a tale of some serious chemical exposure that had led to a sad life-altering condition. We exchanged stories of doctors' visits with no answers and no cures.

There was a desperate hopeless feeling among us. What would happen to us? Why weren't the words "Multiple Chemical Sensitivities" ever mentioned on the news or the television shows? Why was this some kind of "closet" illness? Was there something to be ashamed of? Certainly this condition felt very important to me, and I was not ashamed. Just because the doctors couldn't identify it, didn't mean it should go unnoticed!

People are being hurt in toxic environments and still the doctors debate whether or not this illness is real. As Lynn Lawson states in her book, *Staying Well in a Toxic World,* (I didn't throw it away as the doctor suggested) " . . . many traditional doctors still do not believe that EI/MCS exists. It's not hard to see why. EI/MCS is a usually invisible condition caused by usually invisible substances."[5]

I wondered: When will doctors acknowledge MCS as real and very serious? When will there be a cure?

---

[5] Lawson, Lynn, *Staying Well in a Toxic World* (Chicago, IL: The Noble Press, Inc. 1993), 43.

Chapter 3

ISOLATION

As fall merged with winter, I kept despairing about my lost career. I spent more time being upset about that than I did about my lost health. I missed working each day. My life was empty and boring, with no purpose. By wintertime, I was getting the picture that I was in serious trouble and that my focus should be on regaining my health.

I sat alone each day and wondered how this had happened. I questioned my life and dwelled on all the mistakes that might have made me vulnerable to the injury. I was depressed and I was lonely. It seemed that friends at work had written me off. They perhaps didn't understand what was wrong with me. The phone seldom rang. One friend from school consistently called, but it was painful to hear about all the fun she was having. I could tell she didn't understand when I tried to explain my symptoms. She told me to ignore them and just carry on. She said that's what she would do.

I lived in the past and reviewed my life. I remembered my friends in college. I thought about my junior year abroad in Switzerland. How I had loved skiing! I thought about my music that I loved so much. I had been a singer and a pianist. I had appeared many places. Two years before my injury, I recorded a Christian cassette "Believe, Just Believe." I had sung on television and radio programs. It was such a promising time. Now, all that was over.

Then I reviewed my years as a teacher. I had worked so hard to get a master's degree, attending classes at night. I went all the way into Boston, which was a twenty-five mile trek each way. I had even gone on to earn forty-five credits beyond the master's. There were so many additional workshops where I could learn more and enrich my teaching style. I just worked so hard. For what? . . . to spend each day alone by the open window trying to breathe?

I had to learn about other ways to help my body, because there were no adequate answers from the traditional medical community. The asthma medications I had been placed on were making me sick. I used an inhaler. My throat constricted each time I sprayed the substance into my mouth. The medicine was making me extremely shaky and nervous. I could hardly sleep at night.

David brought me a book called, *Sinus Survival,* written by Dr. Robert Ivker. I was still unable to breathe through my nose, for my sinuses continued to be completely blocked since the injury. Although I could only read the book for about ten minutes at a time before I had reactions, I was able to read long enough to discover a field of medicine called naturopathy. The description presented in the book intrigued me:

> The basic principles of naturopathy are based on the concept that the body is a self-healing organism. The naturopathic physician enhances the body's own nat-

ural immune response through noninvasive measures and health promotion. Rather than treat the symptoms, naturopaths strive to uncover the underlying cause of patient's disease.[1]

In order to learn more, I called the American Association of Naturopathic Physicians in Kirkland, Washington. The man on the phone further explained the concept of naturopathy. A naturopath helps to heal the body using natural methods such as herbs and vitamins. After we talked for a while longer, I became very interested and asked for the name of a naturopath in my area. He said that I was very fortunate because there was an excellent one nearby, in Massachusetts. When I hung up the phone, I called the number he gave me and spoke with the assistant of Dr. Edward Ellis. I made an appointment for the next week. I was encouraged.

I came to my appointment carrying a huge red bag that contained all the medicines I had to have with me in case of emergency. The bag contained sprays, medicines, and an epinephrine pen (an injection I could administer in case of emergency to stop a serious reaction). Dr. Ellis said I would be able to do away with the medicines as well as the bag. I was pleased to hear this, but I had my doubts.

He began by recommending many herbs, instructing me to take them all at once, at full strength. I hesitated, saying that I was very sensitive. Dr. Ellis said that didn't matter, that herbs were very easy to take.

---

[1] **Chapter 3:** Robert Ivker, M.D. *Sinus Survival* (Los Angeles, CA: Jeremy P. Tarcher, Inc. 1992), 196.

That night I did as he said. Within two days, I was in the midst of a reaction. I had a rash on my face, and my breathing was even worse than before. So much for herbs being easy to take!

I didn't want to give up, for I very much needed to get off the asthma medications. I returned to Dr. Ellis and told him of my predicament. He was very understanding. He assured me that there were many herbs we could try. I asked him to go slower. So, to begin with, he recommended two substances. When I had proven I was not reacting to them, I would return to Dr. Ellis, and add other herbs until we had a program.

This worked! With this combination of herbs and vitamins, my lungs became clearer and stronger. There was ease when I breathed, and there also seemed to be much more air in my lungs. It was a wonderful feeling to be able to take a nice deep breath again! I gradually decreased my medication and, within a month, could throw away the red bag! Still, I had to be very careful to breathe only clean air, but I felt much better and my body was calm. During the night, I was able to sleep better. There seemed to be no negative side effects at all.

Later, Dr. Ellis recommended a natural nose drop that began to heal my sinuses. It took months of using these drops, but eventually, I was able to breathe a bit through my nose.

This was my first venture into "alternative medicine." It was a wonderful step and my interest in herbs began and grew from that time.

I also needed to find a solution to my neck and back problems, which continued to be very painful. One of my phone friends, Glenda, recommended Network Chiropractic. This is a form of chiropractic developed by a man named Donald Epstein. It is called

Network because he selected techniques from different forms of chiropractic and combined them into this specific style of chiropractic work. After an analysis of the spine is done, a light touch is applied to remove patterns of stress and release meningeal tension—tension located in the outer sheath around the brain and the spinal chord. The spine becomes free of subluxations, the twisting or stretching of nerves or the tissue surrounding them. As a result of this correction, the nerves are allowed to deliver a clear flow of energy to the body.

Glenda gave me the name of a practitioner, Dr. Deborah Miller. I went to her and she was wonderful. She worked on my spine very gently and my pain was greatly reduced. Throughout my illness, there were flare-ups, but thank goodness I had Deborah to go to for relief. Due to my very high level of sensitivities, medications and painkillers were not an option for me; a natural approach was imperative. I continue to see her and have the highest regard for her. She has a special healing gift and an excellent knowledge of the body.

It was now winter and I continued searching all the time for help. I needed to get well, but there were still no answers. In January, I had an appointment with a holistic doctor in Newburyport, Dr. Kinderlehrer, who specialized in allergies and MCS. He told me that there was no known cure, but that I could try some herbs and some substances to help me detoxify. He said that I was too sensitive to test for allergies, but that I might be able to test for a histamine drop, which I could use to block reactions. He was very compassionate and he believed that this condition was real, but he, too, offered no absolute answers.

I couldn't tolerate the detoxification product. It was disappointing to realize that my system had become so sensitive that even the treatments were intolerable.

February was very difficult. One day, I went to the dentist's for a cleaning. Without thinking, I followed another person. (I have since learned that I must go first before the chair is treated and the room cleaned.) The chair had been treated with a disinfectant. When I sat down, the room started to swirl around. I felt terrible. I didn't say anything and just let the hygienist clean my teeth. By the end of the treatment, I couldn't take any more. I couldn't stay to let the dentist examine my teeth. I just left and tried to drive myself home. I was dizzy and disoriented. I made it home and I became very ill after that for about two weeks. This chemical exposure rendered me even more sensitive. More and more objects, even food odors, seemed intolerable.

One evening, shortly after that, I awoke with nausea and a pounding headache. David and I were concerned. I noticed a strong odor of soap. David figured out that he had put the dishwasher on before we went to bed, which is what he had been doing so that I would not smell the soap. Our bedroom was upstairs and a good distance from the kitchen.

Suddenly, I had developed a sensitivity to our dishwasher soap. Since I was not well enough to experiment with new soaps, we simply had to stop using the dishwasher.

Then a week later, when I went downstairs one Sunday morning, I became ill again. My head throbbed and I felt like I had a flu. It came on suddenly and I was beginning to learn that this was a reaction. We figured out that the smell of perked coffee that my husband loved and made every Sunday was making me sick. That was the last morning he could drink coffee of any type in the house. He already had to read the Sunday paper out in the sun-room due to the ink and the smell of the paper. Now he had to drink his coffee out there as well. I kept losing the ability to tolerate substances one by one.

I even became sensitive to my little den upstairs. It was actually one of our bedrooms, which we had used as a small reading room. It only contained a couch and a chair. The window was located beside the couch, and I had been sitting by this open window every day, even during the winter. It was the only way I was able to breathe enough fresh air while I was inside the house. Being cold had become a constant state since this illness. Comfort didn't seem to be an issue anymore. It was only survival. Ever since this exposure at the dentist's, the open window didn't help. I just gasped for air and felt sick. I had no idea what that was all about. I tried the kitchen. I seemed to be all right in the dining area, so I sat there by a window. This would become my world for a very long time.

Through my network of telephone friends, I learned about a new treatment for allergies which was called EPD, meaning Enzyme Potentiated De-sensitization. I sent for information about this treatment. The information arrived and a name of a doctor in Massachusetts was also included. I made an appointment to see Dr. English.

When I saw Dr. English, we made arrangements to use EPD. I learned that it was a new technique that involved injections. An enzyme in the injections allowed the body to accept the injected substances at a very low dosage. There were many allergens contained in the injection. One shot every other month for two years would help build up a tolerance for the allergens. It sounded wonderful. The only catch was that I had to be off of all asthma herbs before the shot. I had to read a booklet with directions on what to do before, during, and after the shot was administered. It was very complicated.

I agreed to try the shot. Three days before the appointment, I stopped taking my asthma herbs. It was all right for me to be on medications, but not herbs. Dr. English prescribed drugs for me to try. I began taking them, and I started reacting. By the day before the scheduled shot, I had become quite sick. I had gotten another rash, and my breathing was labored. My lungs felt tight and I could only take shallow breaths. That same day I had been exposed to fires burning outside. It was almost spring and people were cleaning their yards, burning leaves and brush. I had never noticed leaves burning before, but this year I reacted with breathing problems. I also began reacting to yet another substance in my house.

That evening, I had a severe reaction that almost took my life. David perceived my emergency—I could get no air. I could not use an inhaler. I was just lying there looking up at him in despair. He very wisely got the histamine drops I had from Dr. Kinderlehrer. He administered two drops under my tongue. They were amazing. Within minutes, I could breathe. My condition improved. I believe that the drops and David had saved my life.

Later that night, I went back on my asthma herbs. The next day I called Dr. English to tell her what I went through. She was disappointed. So was I. I wanted so much to try this promising treatment.

I would just have to look in another direction.

That same week, I was reminiscing about the past while sitting alone in my chair. I was thinking of my special college friends. I decided to call one of them. When I reached her, we talked for a while. I didn't tell her what I was going through. I didn't know where to begin. I just wanted to talk to her. I was so lonely. Then she told me that one of our close friends was extremely ill. She had Chronic Fatigue Syndrome. I was surprised. I got her number and called her.

When she answered, we talked about her illness. She was much improved and working again. She told me about her doctor, Dr. Green, in Connecticut. I was very interested. He used Chinese herbs, homeopathy, and acupuncture. It sounded great. I called him that day and scheduled an appointment.

Because I had had such a strong reaction that Sunday before, I gradually lost the ability to be in the dining room. I had to stay in my bedroom all day and all night. I could do nothing at all now. David felt sorry for me and at night he read me his favorite stories. They were very masculine, but I loved them. They will always be so special to me. His company meant so much. During that one hour, as he read, I felt a sense of security. His presence next to me was very comforting. My mind traveled with his stories, and I didn't have to think about my dismal reality. When he got tired, we would go to bed. Then the fear would return. I had no idea what would happen to me.

That next week, David drove me to Connecticut to see the new doctor. Dr. Green was very confident about his ability to help me. I bought the herbs he recommended on the first appointment and went home very enthusiastic. I began taking the substances in the amount he advised, but by the next day had begun reacting to them. He wanted me to take nine pills a day. The first day, after taking three, my body began to itch all over. I felt sad. How would I ever get well when taking these pills was so difficult for me?

Even though no improvements were made, I would continue to see this doctor for one year. I even became more sensitive, but I had no other place to turn at that time. If Dr. Green had helped my college friend so much, he must be able to help me! I was desperate. Other friends suggested that I might be detoxing, which would explained the increase in sensitivity. So I continued with the treatments.

It was April, seven months after the injury. The weather was turning warm and I couldn't seem to feel excited about this promising time of year. One day I sat by the peaceful Concord River at the Old North Bridge in Concord, Massachusetts. It was so much easier for me to be outside. As I gazed out at the sparkling water, I wondered what was happening to me. My body had once been so strong and my life had been happy. How had I become so frail and thin? Where was I heading? There were so many questions without any answers.

Suddenly, I noticed a woman standing next to me. She was a photographer. Much to my surprise, she asked if she could take my picture because I looked so serene. I hesitantly agreed. As she clicked the camera, I wondered if the photo would ever catch the inner turmoil and the suffering I so expertly hid. This was the last day I would be able to sit outside for an afternoon. After that, my health continued to fail and my activities became more and more restricted.

That same month, I was notified that a hearing was scheduled for my worker's compensation claim. The insurance company had scheduled an appointment for me with a doctor of their choice, Dr. Wyner.

Within minutes of entering his waiting room, I began to react. There were no windows and there were too many odors for me. I kept going outside and coming back in to see if he was ready for me. Finally after an hour and a half, I was informed that he was ready. I was ushered into a small examining room, again with no windows. I asked if there was one with windows. The receptionist said there was not. After waiting for ten minutes, I began to have difficulty with my breathing. I got up and opened the door to the hallway to get some air. The doctor went by, gave me an annoyed look, and shut the door. After waiting a few more moments, I got up and opened it again. I just needed more air. Once again, when the doctor went by, he shut the door. I did not feel well. So, I got up and left the room. I asked the receptionist how much longer it would be before I could see the doctor. She didn't know. I went outside to regain my breathing ability and to clear my head. Finally, after another half hour, the doctor was really ready to see me.

I went back into the stuffy little room. A man with intense eyes and wildly curly hair came into the room and shut the door. I didn't say anything, because he seemed adamant about this door.

Dr. Wyner smiled broadly. I wondered if he was very friendly. As the interview went on, I realized that he was laughing at me. When I described my symptoms, he chuckled. Other times he laughed. I finally mustered enough courage to ask him why he was laughing. He replied, "It's a long story." I asked him to tell it to me. He just shook his head and laughed. "No, it's too long." Then he continued asking questions and he continued laughing at me. Although I tried to convey the seriousness of my illness and how desperately I was trying to survive, he just kept laughing. Under his breath, he kept chuckling and muttering, "It's a long story."

How could a doctor laugh so blatantly at such a terrible time of my life? Even if he didn't believe in MCS, at least he could have some human compassion! I sure would have loved to have heard that "long story!"

Not only did I have to contend with Dr. Wyner's mockery, but I also had to cope with his after-shave lotion! (I had called ahead the day before to request that he please not wear any fragrances.) I tried to sit as far away from him as possible. When he came near, to examine me, I felt very weak and dizzy. I tried to keep my head away from him. I told him I was having difficulty breathing his after-shave lotion. In response, he laughed, saying his was a "special fragrance" that did not cause sensitivities.

In my case it obviously did not work, for I had to take a shower immediately upon arriving home and change all my clothes. I had to launder the ones I had worn at his office. All this had to be done to attempt to remove the "special fragrance" which was making me sick.

Throughout the entire appointment, he seemed amused at every problem I was having. He clearly had no respect for this illness and didn't try to accommodate me by not wearing a fragrance. What a discouraging and exhausting day!

Toward the end of April, I had to appear for my worker's compensation hearing. A group member, whom I knew from the phone network, had recommended my lawyer. Attorney Sands was considered to be a very polite man and he agreed to represent me. That meant a lot.

Appearing in court was a difficult challenge for me. The courtroom was filled with people wearing fragrances. In order to receive my benefits, I had to be present. Nobody assisted me in any way. To avoid the fragrances, I waited for my turn in a small room, alone. Many hours passed.

I realized then that, although the court pays lip service to Environmental Illness, it truly does not understand the condition. Part of the disability for a person with Environmental Illness involves great difficulty being able to be in public buildings. It is extremely hard if no provisions are made. In court, I needed the people present to refrain from wearing fragrances. It would have helped if I had had access to fresh air, perhaps an open window. Also, I should have been scheduled as the first case so that I could leave as soon as possible. Without these provisions, I was actually being asked to perform tasks that were the very nature of my disability. This has to change! Worker's compensation hearings should not involve an obstacle course, so that if the person survives his court appearance, he might receive benefits. Certainly a person confined to a wheelchair would not be required to climb three flights of stairs to appear at a hearing! This would be utterly unfair. So, too, is it totally unreasonable to require a person who reacts severely to the slightest of odors to endure a courtroom full of people wearing strong perfumes and after-shave lotions! New awareness must evolve to change this abusive treatment.

Finally, after hours of waiting, the judge listened to my story. By the time I appeared before him, I was exhausted. My voice was so weak I could hardly speak. With great effort, I tried to explain my serious health problems. He must have felt sorry for me. He said he would grant me partial disability until he heard what the "impartial doctor" who represents his department, the Division of Industrial Accidents, had to say.

As a result of his decision, I received forty-five percent of what I had made as a teacher. Even though I was totally disabled, my lawyer was happy I would receive some benefits. He hadn't prepared my case until the day before, so he apologized to me. He was relieved that we didn't lose. I felt cheated. I was certainly sick enough to deserve total disability. Oh well, there was much to learn about the legal system.

Although my experience in this area was proving very disturbing, I needed to redirect my attention to the living of my daily life. So much was becoming confusing and perplexing. An entirely new education about survival was becoming necessary for me.

Chapter 4

RELEARNING TO LIVE

By the beginning of May, it was very apparent to me that my usual products and habits were no longer suitable or possible for me. Life had become extremely difficult. All my favorite products were becoming intolerable. I had to throw away all my nail polish and perfume. And still I was bothered by the lingering smell of fragrances from my bureau, where perfume bottles had rested for many years. I even had to go through all my drawers and remove the empty perfume bottles from inside; my mother had taught me that they would add a nice scent to the drawers. All my clothes smelled very pretty, but now it was not possible for me to breathe those fragrances. I could not wear any clothes that had been kept in the bureau. I could only wear the clothes in my closet and those stored in other areas.

I threw away my potpourri, which I had kept in little baskets in my house. Before my injury, I was a person who loved fragrances. My house was filled with them. I even bought French and German soaps to put in my closet. I loved stores with perfume counters and would hope that the clothes I bought there would retain their lovely smell when I brought them home. I just loved pretty fragrances.

Suddenly, my world had turned upside down. I couldn't tolerate any smell at all. When my husband washed his hair, I couldn't go near him for hours. Even my own soap and shampoo bothered me. Everything I had used before the injury now made me sick. What was I to do?

When I began to connect with others who had also been chemically injured, I learned about the products available for Environmentally Ill people. There are numerous catalog companies and specialty places where the focus is on safe and chemical-free products. Thank goodness I found them. I could no longer use products from the regular stores. Even worse, I couldn't even go into the stores to purchase them!

I began to live through the catalogs. The only problem was that many of the catalogs were impossible to read. They contained very odorous inks and paper, making the selection of an item quite difficult. Also, more often than not, I would spend money to buy a product and I would not even be able to keep it in the house. I often returned many products or just threw them away. Even the items made especially for chemically sensitive people were extremely difficult for me to be around or use.

At least there were wonderful companies that had excellent products. It was a relief to find a few items I could use and tolerate. Some companies I found helpful were Janice Corporation, Harmony, The Living Source, N.E.E.D.S., Reflections Organic Clothing, and Coastline Products. These names and addresses are included in an appendix at the back of this book. Some of the companies were even considerate enough to make their catalogs readable for sensitive people by using safe paper and ink. They were a pleasure.

Life had gotten to be a challenge. Each product I lost the ability to use caused me a major effort to replace safely. I had to search everywhere for a shampoo. Finally, N.E.E.D.S. made one that was very simple and unscented. I could tolerate it if I used a little bit. Then I searched for a new facial cleanser. I needed one that was fragrance-free. I found a wonderful product made by a company named Annemarie Borlind. This search went on each time I needed a product—even down to a lip balm for the winter. Because I no longer could tolerate my usual brand, I just used Vitamin E. It was very helpful. So much that I used to do and take for granted now required extra effort and was so time-consuming.

I kept throwing away my products. I was very sad to dispose of all my make-up. No more lipsticks, blush, eye make-up, etc.—products that made me feel feminine. I lost them all. I could do nothing with cosmetics. Besides, I didn't have any reason to dress up. I had no life!

Other family members become directly affected when one person is injured and develops Environmental Illness. David's life had to change drastically. He, too, had to change his personal products. He had to use only products that I could tolerate. This was difficult for him. He had a favorite soap he had always used. However, it contained a fragrance, so it had to go. He had to change his brand of shaving cream and he stopped using after-shave lotion. He lost one thing after another. He never complained, but I know it was difficult for him.

He could not do any projects in the house; everything bothered me. We had to change our laundry detergent to an unscented one. He had to take a shower the moment he got home if he had gone to a store or to a meeting. Stores have so many odors and chemicals. All of these lingered on his clothes. It even bothered me if he walked through the room, so sometimes he had to leave his clothes in the garage and come into the house naked. This was so difficult, yet, he never complained—he never smiled either, but he never complained.

We even had to ask our neighbors to help me. We asked them to please not resurface their driveways, because I had to sit by an open window at all times. I could not close the window. If I had to breathe asphalt, I could become very ill. Even when we drove by a construction site on the road, I would take one breath of asphalt and be unable to think or speak for about an hour. Luckily our neighbors were wonderful. I know they had always been responsible about sealing their driveways every year, but not one of them did this year. They really came through for me and I was very grateful.

I still had to contend with the chemical treatments of their lawns for fertilizing or insect control. I could not complain about that as well, but I did call the companies and request that they call me before they came to treat the lawns. Then I would have to close the windows. David would take me for a ride in the car and bring me back home later. I was amazed at how many times people treated their lawns. The companies came about nine times during one season. There were three neighbors who used them. That's twenty-seven applications I had to worry about!

I also had to be vigilant about mosquito spraying by the town. Much to my dismay, I learned that even if I placed myself on the "no spray" list, the company hired by the town to spray could come and fog the entire yard of the property right next door. Thank goodness my direct neighbors were very aware and never requested to be sprayed. I had to call the company three times a week. I got to know the gentleman very well. He was ready for me each time. He would tell me exactly what part of town they were spraying and how close they would come. I don't know what I would have done if a close neighbor had requested to be sprayed. There was really nowhere I could go to be safe. I never realized before how many chemicals are around us all the time. We just do not tune into them if we do not react to them. Even so, they are going into our bodies and we don't even realize it.

Environmental Illness is devastating for those who love you. They see you losing ground and suffering, but there is nothing they can do. My mother could not come near me. She had cigarette smoke on all her clothes because my father smoked. She tried to do so much to accommodate me but nothing worked. She bought a new deodorant, new laundry detergent, and personal products. She tried to buy all unscented products and still I could not tolerate her clothes. I reacted each time she came near. David told her not to give up, but she was so afraid of hurting me with reactions. She finally stopped trying and I could no longer see her. She was heartbroken.

David never gave up, even when he caused me numerous reactions. Sometimes he had to sleep in the other bedroom, for I could not tolerate the smell of something on him. We never knew what I would react to. Our lives were horrible and we had no idea what was going on. There seemed to be little known about this illness and doctors were no help. There were no solutions and I was slowly losing my life.

We had to find our own answers. After months and months of trial and error, we finally got a grip on the lifestyle we needed to live in order to minimize my reactions. We had a strict routine, which many people would find intolerable. Only small chores could be accomplished very carefully. Any dust or disturbance in the air could set off a reaction. Nobody except David could enter our home due to the fragrances on a visitor's clothing or scented personal products. All of my time was spent alone in the dining room, while David watched television or read in the den. We spoke very little. There was no joy in living. We clung to life, and we did what we had to do in hopes that someday some miracle or treatment would return me to my husband as a person and as a wife.

Chapter 5

A DOWNWARD SLIDE

*I*t was now June. I had missed one entire year of school! I would never know my students. Nine months after the injury and I still could not undo the damage caused by two weeks of toxic fumes! What had they done to my body? Meanwhile, I had lived in solitary confinement as if I were being punished for some crime I had committed. I had seen many doctors of all types and still there were no absolute answers. I was constantly getting worse and I was getting more discouraged. What a waste of my life!

My constant quest was to find fresh air. I had never realized before how rare a commodity is clean, fresh air. During the winter months, there was constant smoke from neighborhood fireplaces and I often had to close my window. I could only easily breathe the air in the house for about one or two hours. Then I would check to see if I could open the window to get fresh air. Sometimes I had to drive around to find a spot where the air was fresh and I would sit there with my car window open so that I could breathe. Without clear, fresh air, I would get dizzy and have difficulty thinking. Also, my breathing would be very labored.

I thought that spring would have eased this situation; however, I had been very wrong. It was even worse during the spring. People saw this wonderful time, when the air is so clear and beautiful, as a perfect opportunity to burn leaves and brush in their yards. This smoke was even harder to breathe than the smoke from fireplaces. It was so thick and heavy. It seemed constant. Again, I often had to leave and go somewhere else in my car. I got to know all the rules and regulations. Burning was permitted between the hours of ten and four. So I was dressed and prepared to leave by 10:00 A.M. I was relieved that there was no burning on Sundays. I loved Sundays!

I have really learned just how careless we are about our very precious air supply. Two years before my injury, David and I had traveled to Switzerland, where I had studied during my junior year abroad. We visited a little village near the Matterhorn called Zermatt. When we arrived, we marveled at the different kind of air we were breathing. It was clear, absolutely crystal clear! There were no gas-powered cars allowed in the entire village. Nothing contaminated the air. We couldn't believe the difference. We had never breathed anything like it!

Now, I would have given anything to breathe that pure and healthy air again. I had to work constantly to find clean air, and it was a full-time job!

By June, I was able to use my dining room, having spent one month of seclusion in the bedroom. It was a relief to be able to tolerate this space again. David didn't have to read to me anymore, for I could sit in my chair at the dining room table. It was actually a large room with a kitchen on one end and a dining area on the other. The kitchen was difficult for me because of the smell of the finish on the cabinets. My time limit in that section was only about ten minutes. I could at least prepare something to eat and then return to the dining area. There was very little around me. The table was made of glass and the chairs were wood with soft, beige cloth cushions. Two very long windows were on my right—they looked out upon our pretty yard and the street. We lived on a cul de sac, so not many cars went by. My view was very peaceful; it consisted of a large expanse of grass interspersed with perennial flower gardens and shrubbery. David and I had planted every item in our yard over the years. Each plant and flower held its own special memory. Now, as I gazed upon them, I saw more and more weeds collecting. The grass was getting bare from lack of attention. Still I felt comforted by this view of my beloved yard.

Mounted on the wall, directly across from me, was a painting of an ocean harbor with four small boats tied to the pier. It was a picture that I would get to know very well over the next few years!

My sole companion during those long lonely days was a wooden clock with little gold Roman numerals, which my mother's friend had crafted for me as a wedding present. It hung on the wall to my left between the kitchen and dining area. As it ticked, I would watch the hands move slowly by each hour— ever so slowly. This constant ticking kept me company all day long. It was the only sound in my life. Sitting alone in my chair and listening to my clock became my life for a very long time. Finally, at the end of each interminably long day, when evening arrived, I could go to bed, go to sleep, and escape the misery. Oh, how I loved to go to bed!

In late June, I received a notice from the Division of Industrial Accidents, notifying me that I had to go to an appointment to see a doctor, regarding my worker's compensation claim. I called the leader of the Massachusetts support group for the chemically injured to tell her who I was being sent to see. She had become my telephone friend. She was a very intelligent former teacher who had also been injured in her school. She knew of this doctor and said that she would put me in touch with another group member, who had gone to see him.

The next day, a man named Brian called. He was very friendly, but he related a tale that dismayed me. He said that this skinny little doctor, who did not believe in MCS, had caused him to lose all his benefits. Brian lived alone and had no one to support him. The doctor knew this, and still he called Brian's condition by some other name, a name he would also use for mine, and destroyed his chances for any compensation. My lawyer also represented Brian.

After I hung up with Brian, I called Attorney Sands immediately and asked, "Why are you allowing me to be sent to Dr. Kane when you know from Brian's letter that he doesn't believe in MCS?" My voice was shaky and I felt nervous. I continued. "How can I possibly prove that I have a condition when the doctor comes to the exam believing that it doesn't even exist! It is impossible and unfair."

My lawyer spoke in his usual calm voice. He said, "Don't worry. Your case is very strong. The facts are very clear about the onset of the illness from the roofing work. You have an excellent career record and you are very sincere. Anyone can see how sick you are." He continued to reassure me.

Still, I was trembling. "Can't we do anything about this unfair treatment?"

He considered quietly, "Well I could request that your own medical records be considered in the decision."

This surprised me. "What do you mean? Aren't they going to be part of my case?"

He replied, "Not usually. Only the 'impartial doctor's' report is considered."

Now I became very worried. "The impartial doctor doesn't believe in MCS! How can I possibly win!" I felt a sinking feeling inside. It was very clear to me that matters were stacking up against me. Even the smooth voice of my attorney was frightening me. This was my life they were all playing with!

Attorney Sands assured me that he would work on it, but I was nervous. He ended with, "Don't worry, you'll be all right even with an unfavorable report from Dr. Kane. The facts are there to support you. You will have to go through with the exam."

When I arrived, the doctor was very cold and aloof. He spoke sternly and did not smile. David asked if he could accompany me for the interview. The doctor refused. He said evenly and curtly, "No, you wait here," indicating a chair outside the door.

Following him into a small, cramped room, I looked immediately for a window and was relieved to see one. I asked him if he would please open it for me. He looked at me strangely, but obliged.

He began his questioning and I related my life's predicament to him. "I am having a very difficult time surviving. I am spending most of my day outside, because I am just not able to be in my home. I can't seem to breathe inside and I feel sick and tired. The only room I can use during the day is my dining area." My hands were trembling and I felt weak. Hearing the actual words as I described my life was extremely upsetting to me. The reality of my dismal predicament was beyond my comprehension.

He listened patiently. At one point, a cool breeze blew in the window. He looked annoyed. He got up and promptly closed the window. He said, "That's enough of that!"

I was upset. This was my air supply. I should have spoken up, but I didn't want to get him angry. He held all the power and I felt like I was at his mercy. He would decide in this one hour if I deserved any compensation, perhaps for the rest of my life!

My own doctors, who had cared for me for almost a year now, would be ignored. This realization made me feel like a victim once again. The system seemed so unfair. My life had been ruined by the roofing fumes, and now I was being treated like this!

So I struggled to breathe and think throughout the interview. When it ended, I rushed to another window in his waiting room and opened it. The fresh air was such a relief. I caught my breath, and tried to regain my strength. I felt weak, dizzy, and extremely tired.

From my previous medical records, he noticed that I had lost a great deal of weight. I had, in fact, lost about twenty pounds and had been thin before the injury. He questioned me about this and seemed a little concerned. However, later when I received his report, he had written the same opinion as he had for Brian. According to him, I had some strange condition, which he termed Multiple Somatic Complaint Syndrome. None of my treating physicians, whose files he had reviewed, had given me that diagnosis. He apparently made it up. His report said that I was indeed totally disabled, and that it had begun at the time of the roofing fumes. But, according to him, that particular injury should have ended three months later, on December 31, 1994. Since it didn't end and I was still disabled, my present condition must not be related! How was I to reason with that logic?

The report emphasized his belief that there is no such illness as "Multiple Chemical Sensitivities." He wrote:

The symptoms currently described by Ms. Smith have been increasingly labeled by some persons with the term 'multiple chemical sensitivities.' This syndrome is not explained by the current principals of toxicology and immunology nor allergy, and important and prominent medical groups in this country have criticized and rejected its existence as an organic disease . . .

The paper continued on and on, attempting to negate the existence of my illness—just as in Brian's report! So I was being examined by a man who didn't treat or understand MCS. He didn't even believe in the condition!

I could only hope that the judge would be intelligent and see how biased this man was.

That summer was the worst of my life. I became light sensitive, which is also called photophobia. It happened rather suddenly one week. I had been spending most of my time outdoors, attempting to breathe more freely, but one day my eyes started seeing dots of light when I looked at the sky. Then I started to feel very sick. My head ached and I felt like I had the flu. I was nauseous and shaky. I went inside to lie down. I had no idea what had happened to me. It took hours to feel well again. The next day I went outside again, only to experience the same symptoms after ten minutes! I was confused. I came inside and had to recover. Each day I tried to go outside and tried to sit in different locations, thinking that maybe there was a plant or flower that was causing this problem; however, nothing seemed to work. I was getting so sick! Finally, one evening, I went outside to sit. Nothing happened to me. I was fine. I became very concerned.

The next day, I called Doctor Kinderlehrer. He said it sounded like photophobia, which meant that I was sensitive to the light! How could this happen? I was stunned. Could it be possible to be sensitive to *light?* Sunshine had always been so special to me. It made me feel wonderful. Now I was sensitive to it! What about being outside to breathe better? Was I only able to be inside where I felt terrible? All these thoughts ran through my mind. I was so frightened. This illness seemed to take away each thing that I loved.

I could not even step outside during the day. I had to wear sunglasses in the house! I could only go out at 7:30 at night. I felt as if I were in prison. My health failed seriously at this point. My body became very weak and frail and I began losing weight again. My head ached most of the time. How do you avoid light! Essentially I was having a reaction all day!

My heart developed arrhythmia, but I was even too sensitive to wear a monitor for the doctor. My blood pressure dropped to below 90/60 most of the time. This made me very tired and feeble. Getting up from a chair required a major effort.

Each day as I weighed myself, the scale reflected that another pound had been lost. During this time, I lost ten pounds, which meant that I had lost a total of thirty pounds since my injury!

My family recognized that I was in serious trouble. David and my mother must have talked and decided that I needed constant supervision. Mom took leave from her job and informed me that she was moving in with me for one month. She figured that if she moved in completely, her clothes would lose their smoky odor and she would be safe for me to be near. I was grateful because I was very sick, but I was also nervous about her coming into my home. When she arrived at my house, I developed flu-like symptoms almost immediately. The smoke odor was strong to me even though she had washed all her clothes. She stayed in the guestroom and didn't come near me for an entire day. The next day, it got a bit easier to be near her. We were so relieved.

She decided that I needed to keep my mind working, so, she tried different things for us to do. The only activity I could tolerate was watching her play solitaire. I could not actually handle the cards (I reacted to them), but I was able to watch her. So, she played and played. I don't know how her hands could keep it up for so long!

Then she got the bright idea that we could listen to books on tape. I really didn't care what we did. She went to the library and brought back different stories. We began to listen each day, just a little. Mom played the tapes outside my bedroom door; I had to be away from the tape recorder because of the plastic. I would just lie there and listen for as long as I could. At first I resisted; I was not interested in anything. Then, gradually, I got a little interested in the story. Since I had to stay in my darkened bedroom during the hours between noon and four, I was glad to have something I could do for a bit of that time.

One day in the late afternoon, my mother was watching me just sit aimlessly in a chair. She asked me if I had ever considered writing. I complained that this was impossible because I could not hold a pen, use a computer, or a typewriter. She thought and thought. Then, she came over to me at the table and handed me an old pencil and a pad of paper. She said, "You can hold a pencil, can't you?" I said that I thought so. She continued, "Then write with this. Just write!"

I was still negative. I asked her what I should write. She said that I might try a children's story. I considered this idea. I could just try it. So, I began. I had always made up little stories and loved to write.

I worked all afternoon and into the night. I wrote my first of many children's stories. This kept my mind busy. When I was finished I read her my story. She was genuinely impressed. She said I should continue to write, and that someday I might have them published. I laughed. She was a wonderful mother! I continued to write all through my illness. I now have many children's stories written. Perhaps, I may have them published someday.

By the end of July, I was close to giving up and my family knew it. My mother virtually kept me alive that summer. She kept talking to me and relating stories about what was going on out in the world. Even when I told her I didn't care, she continued anyway.

To help me get through the days without despairing, I had to put a star on the calendar at the end of each day I had made it through. I knew I had to keep myself going, so I strove for each star. I still have that calendar and it reminds me of the courage it took to survive.

My father lectured me over the phone and told me to work on things and not to die. He said I couldn't let myself die. My mother just kept me going so that I wouldn't die. She sat by my bed on days when my heart was laboring to beat, and she played and played solitaire when I could get up and get dressed. It was a terrible summer, but I survived, and I went on. My mother was the one who really got me through.

I still have the deck of worn-out cards and I feel the love of my mother each time I handle them. I'm afraid to use them these days, for they are falling apart. I keep them as a tribute to a wonderful mother.

By that fall, a whole year after the injury, I had become sensitive to sound and could not listen to the radio, music, or tapes anymore. My world was growing smaller and I was becoming more and more frightened.

I also was having difficulty when I washed my clothes. The laundry detergent was now bothering me, even though it was without fragrance or dyes. I looked everywhere for another soap I could use. Then I learned about laundry discs, which are small plastic discs with tiny ceramic balls inside. They change the ionic composition of the water so that dirt and other matter are pulled out of the clothes. This seemed like a good answer. I ordered a package. It was a relief to learn that I could tolerate them. Still, each time I washed an item, I was nervous that I would not be able wear it when I went to put it on.

Even with the laundry discs, there was still a chemical odor on the clothes after they were laundered. At times this smell seemed strong. In an effort to figure out what it could possibly be, I called the manager of the town water department. The gentleman informed me that they had added a "tiny" amount of chlorine to the water, but that nobody *should* be able to notice it. Well I had! They just didn't know what it was like to be very sensitive.

In October, when we turned the heat on for the first time, I became completely confused and disoriented. I couldn't think or speak! My husband was home and saw my rapid decline. He turned the heat off and within two hours, I had regained my ability to speak. Feeling confused about this new symptom, I called Dr. Kinderlehrer. He called it a brain fog. I had always had an excellent mind, and I was now afraid that it was being injured. Our stove gave off gas fumes, so I stopped using it. We had gas hot-air heat and I decided that I would have to just turn it off. I wore three sweaters, two pairs of pants, three pairs of socks, and two pairs of gloves. I was *so* cold!

We began the search for a safer way to heat our home. This seemed like an almost impossible task, since almost everything I tried to do bothered me. Finally, we conferred with a building consultant named John Bowers. His wife, too, had MCS, and he had dealt with all these issues. He gave us some helpful suggestions. We decided to try a type of electric heater called "Intertherm™." The heaters warm at a low temperature so that they do not burn up dust or carpet fibers. They have virtually no odor.

We ordered one heater. When it arrived, we put it out in the sunroom and turned it on to burn off any new smell it might have. It was getting very cold in our house. It was November and I still refused to turn on the heat. I needed so desperately to preserve my mind.

My father kept advising me to turn the heat on so the pipes would not freeze, but I was insistent. He just didn't understand the illness, saying it was my imagination. He was very worried and tried to protect me in the best way he could, but I had to stand my ground. After all, I had a friend with MCS who had had to move into a tent when she became allergic to her home. If she could survive in a tent in the middle of winter, I could stand being in a cold house until we found another source of heat.

Finally in November, the odor from the new Intertherm™ heater was burned off. We had it installed in the dining area. The next morning the room felt warm. It was wonderful. However, initially I could not be in the room when the heat was turned on. So, first, I would heat the room while I stayed in my cold bedroom. Then I would go to the dining area, turn the heater off and sit there. When I got cold, I would repeat the cycle. It was inconvenient, but it was a relief to get some warmth. Finally, by December, I could stay in the room while the heat was on. Heaven!

We bought another Intertherm™ and another until we had heat in some rooms downstairs and eventually in our bedroom. It was a very gradual process, for we had to burn-off each heater for two weeks, and then install it into the house. We had to be very careful so that I would not become sensitive to them. But, thank God, I did not, and we did keep minimally warm that winter.

In November, I had begun acupuncture treatments. I needed to try something else to stimulate my health. The first few treatments seemed to help, but gradually, I became intolerant of the work. I would have terrible neck and back pain after each session. I had to go to Dr. Deborah Miller, my chiropractor, the day after an acupuncture treatment to help me recover. Still, I kept trying. After a couple of months, having made no progress, I discontinued acupuncture.

By Christmas, things had gotten worse. I was trying on a pair of cotton pants that I had not worn before. I breathed the particles of fabric as I was putting them on. I started coughing and choking. After that, I became allergic to cotton! When I realized this, I became so frightened that I shook myself to sleep that night. How would I survive in New England without clothes? What would happen to me? The next day, I tried to wear my cotton sweaters. I had great difficulty breathing and my throat felt like the fibers were stuck in it. I kept taking off one sweater and trying another. Still the reactions persisted. I was so scared. What was I going to do? David tried to calm me and he brought me clothes to try. He gave me an old gray sweatshirt of his and I tried it on. It was okay! Then I found an old pair of gray corduroys. They too were fine. So, finally I had an outfit. Little did I know then that I would wear only that outfit for the next two years!

After taking a shower later that day, I found that I could not even use a towel to dry myself off. I could not breathe. So, from that point on, I had to drip-dry after showering. I felt so cold!

This turn of events terrified me. Now I was in a mess. Cotton was the only material that I had been able to wear since my injury. Before this latest reaction, I had a very limited supply of clothes I could tolerate. At least I had a few sweaters and a few pairs of pants. Now I was down to one outfit. What would happen if I became allergic to that? My fear was beyond anything I had ever experienced. I shook myself to sleep and awoke shaking in the morning. I prayed desperately to God. I needed Him to please rescue me from this horrible situation. I asked how this had ever happened to me. I had no idea something like this could happen to anyone. I begged God to help me find a way to stop being allergic to my clothes. Still the agony went on, day after day. David could not even touch me on the shoulders to calm me—we had to be careful so that the fibers did not go into the air and make me allergic to my last outfit.

Life was horrible. To go to a doctor, I had to be blindfolded and driven by David. The light was very painful for my eyes. This was one of the saddest developments of all, for I had always loved the sunshine!

David had to do all the housework; I could not tolerate any dust or particles in the air. If he vacuumed the upstairs, I could not go up for eight hours. He vacuumed downstairs when I went to bed in the evening. By the next morning, I could go safely downstairs. David had to take a shower before coming to bed so that I would not react to the dust that was on him. He did the laundry because of my sensitivity to clothes. Since we had a gas stove that we couldn't use, he had to cook on a gas grill outside. We were struggling to survive and still I had no answer of how to get well. Doctors just kept shaking their heads and saying they were sorry for me.

David had become exhausted. He never smiled anymore. This was quite a drastic change for him. Before my injury, he had always enjoyed relating funny stories; he loved to see me laugh. David is an optical engineer. His intelligence constantly amazed me, and yet he was a very regular and friendly person. He was tall, strong, and wonderful. One year prior to my chemical exposure, he had been laid off and decided to start his own optics company. It was very small and he ran it himself. This placed great pressure on him; he had to work many more hours to build the company in order to pay the bills. After my injury, his hours were filled with worry and stress. During the day, he couldn't turn the heat on because he did not have enough money; he worked in one small cold room with a little electric heater beside him. After working twelve hours a day at his new struggling company, he would return home to take care of me.

One sad evening, after we had eaten, he wearily looked at me and said, "Sometimes, I wish that I could change places with you. I know you are suffering and your life is terrible, but so is mine. I just hope I can make it through this." He saw the tears in my eyes and he continued. "Nothing matters anymore. All I care about is you getting well."

This was the first time he had expressed these feelings, and I was acutely aware of the huge effect this injury had had on his life. How terrible I felt to know that this illness had ruined his life as well! If only I could heal and give David some hope.

During this time I prayed constantly to God for help. I couldn't imagine continuing to live this way. I was suffering so! I had lost my rosary beads, so I didn't pray to the Holy Mother at all. Desperately, I begged God to cease this agony. My prayers were weak and sorrowful pleas for His assistance. There seemed to be no way out!

In the midst of this, I had to go to the laughing doctor again for the insurance company. I arrived with David and waited outside in the car. David came to get me when the doctor was ready. We thought that maybe the doctor would not laugh at me if David were present. The appointment did go a little better. I was so sick, but, even so, the doctor was rather mocking. When I asked him to please open the door, he asked me why. I tried to explain that I needed fresh air. He smirked and said that there was "air" all around me. I then tried again to explain that I needed fresh air. He asked caustically, "Cold air?" Then I stated, "No, fresh air." He continued, "Cold air?" I again stated, "No, fresh air." This went on. My husband could take it no longer. He emphatically stated, "She needs fresh air, not cold, *fresh!*"

The doctor ceased that round of questions. I was having great difficulty speaking, for my mind was affected by the lack of air. I remember telling him that I had no life and that I was suffering. He smiled again and said curtly, "You have a life. It's a life." This man amazed me. He was so cruel.

During our ride home, David said, "I can't believe that man graduated medical school! What are they teaching? He didn't even know the difference between fresh air and cold air! He was making fun of you! What a stupid man!"

Clearly David was tired of the cruelty to which I was being subjected. He tried so hard to take care of me and he needed a little cooperation from others. Yet there seemed to be none!

It appeared that abuse and ridicule were going to be part of the effort to obtain my benefits. It was all

I had experienced and I was getting beaten down. My body was so weak and tired that I just tried to ignore the foolish hired doctors. My life was at stake here, and my focus had to be on that issue most of all.

However, this appointment did give David a long-lasting joke with me. Any time I would say to him, "I need fresh air," he would reply, "Cold air?" I would then say, "No, fresh air!" He would answer, "Cold air?" At first I did not laugh, but later it got to be sort of funny. We still say it once in awhile.

In January, fifteen months since I'd been injured, I had to appear in court in Boston for another worker's compensation hearing. This was very difficult for me. David accompanied me, because I was still needing a blindfold to shut out the light. We were in court all day. I told the judge about my life and he listened silently. It was probably hard for him to believe. It certainly was hard for me to grasp. The day in the court made me very sick physically. I did not recover for several weeks. I became extremely tired and even more sensitive.

In February, I appeared in court once again to finish telling the sad story of my injury. This time my husband had to testify. He described the misery of our lives. He explained that he, too, was struggling; life was very hard for him as well.

Even my principal was summoned. He testified that I had been a very excellent teacher and confirmed that the fumes were present in the school. He agreed that I had been badly affected by them. He tried to help me receive my benefits. I appreciated his efforts.

I heard the next week that the principal had gone back to school and told others that I had looked terrible and had aged so much. I think he finally realized what I was going through. Up until then no one from school had contacted me to ask me how I was doing. This had saddened me. I had hoped that someone would care and maybe even *apologize.*

That winter, I finally gave in and officially applied for Accidental Disability Retirement. An agreement in my retirement plan stated that if I were injured at work, I would be entitled to a certain portion of my pay as a retirement. I had to see three doctors on their medical panel. If two out of three agreed that I was disabled as a result of a work experience, then the board could grant me my pension. I certainly qualified for this, but it was very difficult for me to apply. I could not really accept that I would never return to my once-cherished profession. Doctors and family members tried to talk sense into me and convinced me that I needed to apply. Because I had only been allowed to pay into the Massachusetts Teacher's Retirement Plan, I could not receive any Social Security disability benefits. So, without my teaching pension, I would have nothing else.

Spring was approaching. It had now been a year and a half since my initial exposure to the roofing fumes. I was still struggling to survive. I could only be in one room of my home during the day and my bedroom at night. Every other room in my home made me sick. I could not go outside. I could not listen to music. I could not read a book, or watch television. I could only talk on a speaker telephone for ten minutes at a time, because I was allergic to plastic, and the sound was too difficult for me. I was all alone all day in a chair, in a dark room with no sound, while the clock ticked away my life.

In the words of Dr. Robert Sampson, in the book he co-authored with Patricia Hughes, *Breaking Out of Environmental Illness:*

Imagine a world where everything around you makes you sick. Your food, clothing, and shelter produce symptoms that may affect any organ in your body. Even low levels of chemicals that do not affect other people trigger reactions in you. Your life becomes a constant struggle to protect yourself from toxins that are everywhere around you. This is the world of someone with Environmental Illness.[1]

This had become my life.

----

[1] **Chapter 5:** Robert Sampson, M.D. and Patricia Hughes, B.S.N. *Breaking Out of Environmental Illness* (Santa Fe, NM: Bear & Company, 1997), 11.

Chapter 6

THE BLESSED MOTHER HOLDS MY HAND

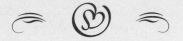

*I*t was March of 1996, one and a half years since the injury. This was a cold and tiring month. The days were dragging on. My life was filled with despair. It was time to come to terms with God. My spirituality was enduring a great test. It had been unchallenged when life was easy. However, now I seriously needed help and I felt that God had abandoned me. My prayers were of desperation and fear, not of love.

The question I often asked was, "Why, God, has this happened to me?" It all did not make any sense.

All my life I had been a Catholic, attending church on Sundays and singing in the choir. It was a deep and meaningful experience. Sometimes I had questions about the teachings, but I felt a profound love each time I sang to God.

Two years before my injury I had recorded a cassette of Christian songs, some of which I had written. The songs had been very well received. I had appeared on television shows and had been a guest on the radio. My music was being featured on many Christian programs.

Soon after this, the fumes destroyed my life. Why had God let this happen to me? Why hadn't He protected me? I felt I didn't deserve to suffer like this. From that point on, I didn't pray with all my heart; I didn't believe that God was listening.

One day, in late March, a package arrived for me. My mother's friend Carol, a devout Catholic, had been our spiritual teacher, always talking of God and His role in our lives. My mother had made her acquaintance at work; they had remained friends through the years. She was praying for me and very concerned about what had happened. She sent me some tapes about the Blessed Mother.

I listened to the tapes very softly, for it hurt my ears to listen. The tape was very beautiful, and I began to feel the deep need to pray to the Blessed Mother. Finally I couldn't listen any more. I remembered that I had lost my rosary beads many months before. I had casually looked around the house for them, but to no avail. Now I needed them! I prayed seriously for the first time. I said something like, "Please Blessed Mother, find my rosary beads for me. I can't find them. I need to pray to you!"

Right after my prayer, I got up and began to search for the beads. Still unable to locate them, I gave up.

The next morning, Sunday, I got up and opened my bureau drawer to obtain my clothing. As I began to close the drawer, a strong, beautiful fragrance of flowers engulfed me. Usually, being so sensitive made me detest the smell of flowers, but this time it was wonderful. I quickly reopened the drawer to see what was happening. Automatically, I placed my hand under the clothes directly onto a box. When I pulled out the case, I saw immediately that it was my rosary beads!

I sat on my bed and thanked the Blessed Mother. I felt her presence everywhere. I knew from that moment on that she was with me. Each day thereon I prayed a rosary to her. I felt she was near and that she would help me through this injury. I was not alone anymore.

From that point, whenever I had a reaction, which was often, I would turn to Mother Mary and ask her to help me find the reason. Soon after my prayer, the answer would come. I needed her.

One terrible evening, she again came into my life. Ever since my exposure to the fumes, something had happened to my neck and back. The right side of my body seemed to be injured. Every couple of weeks or so, I would suddenly develop a horrible pain in my neck, which permeated my body. I would be nauseous and dizzy. My face ached and my head throbbed. I felt sick all over. Lying down was agony; the pain would worsen. I usually would see my chiropractor, Deborah Miller, and she would help me relieve the pain. This evening the pain came suddenly. It was severe. I felt so ill that I stayed sitting in the bathroom—I thought I was going to vomit.

I called Deborah Miller. It was around 9:00 in the evening, and I hadn't wanted to bother her, but I couldn't bear the pain any longer. She wasn't home, so I left a message. I told her she could call me at any time; I wasn't going to go to sleep that night with that kind of pain. I couldn't take any aspirin, or any other medicines; I was sensitive to them.

I went into the bathroom to wait for her call. Rocking gently on the floor, I began to sing to the Blessed Mother. I found I was actually writing a new song. Words came to me, and melody as well. I sang softly:

Hold my hand Blessed Mother. Hold my hand.
Hold my hand Blessed Mother. Hold my hand.

I am weary and I do not understand.
Hold my hand Blessed Mother. Hold my hand.

I cannot see the light beyond the trees.
I cannot feel the warmth beyond the breeze.
I cannot hear the laughter beyond the heavy
  tears.
Hold my hand Blessed Mother. Calm my fears.

Hold my hand Blessed Mother. Hold my hand....

As the verses developed automatically, I continued to sing. When the song was finished, I sat still. I thanked the Blessed Mother for the beautiful song. I thought that someday when I was well, I could record that as a tribute to her. But even more wonderful—the excruciating pain was gone! Completely gone!

Then Deborah Miller called. I listened to her instructions on how to work on my neck myself, but I didn't need to do it—the pain had been completely resolved. Once again the Blessed Mother had lovingly rescued me. I went peacefully to sleep that night and felt protected.

This spiritual connection to the Divine Mother brought me such peace and hope. Along with her constant company, I also developed other new relationships that encouraged a sense of security and comfort. These dear caring individuals who reached out to share with me became known as my "telephone friends." As I relate their stories, you will see there are many wonderful people, isolated in their homes, attempting to recover.

Chapter 7

CONNECTIONS

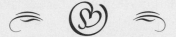

As my illness set in, I became more and more lonely. I needed company and yet I couldn't tolerate people near me. It is a great challenge when one has Environmental Illness to remain connected to the outside world and yet not be bothered by reactions. Being with my mother and David was a constant struggle that required extraordinary measures. My only other contacts were dear and loving friends who reached out to me on the telephone. I share with you now the precious connections that kept me going during the long and lonely duration of Environmental Illness.

My mother and I were very close, but I couldn't have her in my home. If she visited for just one day, the smell of my father's cigarette smoke on her clothes made me sick. Mom made many changes, and still I couldn't have her near me. Only the one-month visit, when she helped sustain me through the summer, was manageable. As soon as she returned to her home and my father's cigarette smoke, it was not possible for her to visit me again. I missed her so. I didn't even try to see anyone else; it was too complicated for me to be safe around another person. Thankfully, I was well around my husband. He was extremely careful. He meant so much to me. I saw him only at night around 7:00—he now had to work many more hours since I had lost my career—even Saturdays. So my time with him was limited and I was *very very* lonely.

My only lifeline to the world was my telephone. I was not able to use a regular phone; direct sound next to my ear continued to cause pain. A speaker-phone eased this problem. I could only use it for about ten minutes before the sound began to hurt, but I did have ten minutes at a time.

The sicker I got, the fewer phone calls I received from friends I had known prior to the injury. They became more and more skeptical and grew distant. It was difficult for them to understand this mysterious illness. I was ignored by nearly everyone and it seemed that nobody cared. Each phone call was so precious to me, and yet I received so very few.

The connections I gradually made with my new telephone friends sustained me. Before this illness, I had no idea of the suffering and the chronic illnesses with which people were coping.

As word began to spread of my injury, other suffering people were kind enough to call and reassure me. Some of them belonged to the group called, "Massachusetts Association for the Chemically Injured" (M.A.C.I.). I had joined the group three months after I was injured. Even though I chose not to attend the actual meetings, members heard of my plight and called. They shared their stories of chemical injuries. It surprised me to hear of such intelligent people being so badly injured! I was amazed that I had never heard of this illness before it happened to me. There seemed to be so many people who were dealing with it. Most of them were confined to their homes and struggling, as I was, to find an answer.

I was extremely impressed with their bravery to be able to go on each day. Enduring a serious illness requires such fortitude and courage.

Other people who heard of my plight were not members of the group. Word had spread through a type of network among those who were ill. These individuals too, were wonderful people who had chronic illnesses that doctors simply could not treat. They were attempting to find answers. This sick and struggling community opened up to me with warmth and kindness. I will always thank them for this caring; I was not alone anymore!

I include here stories of some of my dear "telephone friends."

Glenda was the wife of my dentist. When my dentist had heard about my illness, he informed Glenda, who called me. This phone call was the beginning of a long and close friendship. I liked her immediately. We were in sync. She related her story of struggling for her health for over twenty years. She had extensive food allergies. Doctors she had gone to didn't recognize her problem when she went to them. They placed her on medications, making matters worse. At one point, she had lost so much weight that she was practically bedridden. She could only eat carrots, parsley, quinoa, fish, and seaweed. Her husband was always trying to find a new and exotic meat for her to eat. He attempted to find new foods to which her body had not developed an allergy. But, eventually, she became sensitive to even these foods. She just couldn't eat! How frightening this must have been.

Her best answer came from Network Chiropractic. These treatments improved her health for five years. Then, one summer she attended a week-long energy workshop. By the end of the course, her body was out of balance; she had become light sensitive. Along with this, she had become very sensitive to any type of energy work. She could no longer be treated with Network Chiropractic. Vitamins and herbs were not possible due to her food intolerances. She could not benefit from any type of healing work at all. When I met her she was at this point. Twenty years of trying to heal and still no better!

If I could describe Glenda, I would call her a humanitarian. She tried to help everyone, as well as herself. The moment she heard about a new treatment, she was on her personal "Internet." She called all her friends and her network of ailing people. She couldn't enjoy a healing technique unless others were benefiting from it as well.

Another wonderful attribute about Glenda was a special gift she had developed while using Network Chiropractic. She had become a talented portrait artist. Her graceful portraits captured the person exactly. She read the expression and conveyed the essence of the person. The paintings were wonderful. She was not chemically sensitive so she was able to tolerate the water-soluble paints. This artwork was truly a pleasure for her and a valued gift for others.

Glenda never gave up hope. Together we searched for answers to our problems. We talked each day and constantly discussed our healing. There was nothing she wouldn't do to get better. However, her options had become extremely limited.

Eventually she and I followed similar healing paths and she has improved greatly.

It is said that out of sad times, we are given special gifts. I would have to say that my friendship with Glenda is one of the gifts of this illness. I do not know how I would have gotten through the long and lonely days without her kindness and her love.

Melany was a member of M.A.C.I., the support group I joined. Although I never actually attended the meetings, I got to know her by phone. She had been a nurse for over thirty years. She had been exposed to a wax-stripping chemical one long day in the hospital while she was attempting to work. All day she had breathed the chemicals. By the end of the day, she had a terrible headache and had felt extremely ill. Her sensitivities began after that and progressively intensified until they became very serious. She eventually became sensitive to wood and could no longer reside in her home. Her doctor advised her to move into a tent in the yard. Imagine, a fifty-year-old woman having to live in a tent! She had no choice. For the three months until her sensitivity subsided, she stayed in a tent. It was winter in New England!

If I could describe her in one word, it would be "courageous." She never complained about what she had to do. Her dauntless bravery was my inspiration and my strength. By observing her determination, I was compelled to trudge forward in the face of many obstacles. Her favorite quote was, "You just do what you have to do to get through this!"

Melany utilized many healing modalities. She bought a sauna for her home, had acupuncture treatments, went for massages, and had Enzyme Potentiated Desensitization (EPD) injections. She took numerous herbs and vitamins. She was determined to get over this illness.

Due to the sudden deterioration in their financial status, Melany and her husband were required to sell their home. They purchased a much smaller one in a neighboring town.

After three years of healing work and many lifestyle changes, Melany was making much progress. She was feeling better and living in her recently purchased home. Then, sadly, something happened. Melany relapsed for no understandable reason, and she became very ill again. She is now struggling to heal and her spirits are very low. She developed new sensitivities and had to move from the second home. Once again, she was forced to sell another home. This led her to rent a small cottage from her sister where she felt fairly safe.

We talk every day and I am trying to encourage her. It is hard to know what to say during this very sad time. She was my healing friend and now she must begin again. Melany has been an example of such immense courage that I am confident she will come through this latest setback and feel even stronger as a result of her efforts.

As I look back upon my darkest days, I am extremely grateful that I had a role model as brave as Melany.

Joan was the head of M.A.C.I. She was exposed to pesticides while she had been a teacher. After twenty-three years, she had to leave her profession. Although it had been nine years since her injury, she had not recovered from her loss. Even the mention of her career caused her immense sadness.

Now, her whole life revolved around her mother and the support group. She was dedicated to encouraging people to get together and share their experiences, helping us all to know that we were not alone. She did a fine job.

At one point, I became concerned because I never heard her speak of total healing. She believed that she was permanently damaged and that she could never heal completely. At first I listened to her, but as I progressed, I knew that I needed to be more positive if I expected my body to respond. Our friendship continued, but I was careful not to discuss our theories of healing; they began to differ quite dramatically.

Recently and very sadly, Joan lost her mother. Now Joan is all alone. I hope she will be all right—they were very close. Joan has helped so many people cope with MCS. I hope she will be able to help herself heal from this deep loss.

Brian was also in our group. He was very sad and discouraged. He had worked at a company as a controller for seven years. His office was in a moldy area and he had begun to feel ill. Gradually over time, his health deteriorated and he developed MCS.

Finally, his wife left him and he was forced to sell his home. He lost all his worker's compensation benefits because he was assigned to a doctor who didn't believe in his condition—the same doctor to whom Melany and I had been sent. I guess this was a little bond we all shared with one another. However, Brian had no one to assist him financially, so he essentially became homeless. He was placed on public assistance and had to move in with his elderly parents. Two years after that, his parents moved into elderly housing and Brian was once again left homeless.

Most of the time, Brian was despondent and complained about his plight. I felt sorry for him. I was so lucky to have my husband to help me through the illness. Dealing with Environmental Illness alone requires so much fortitude and courage.

Brian went to different practitioners and never really made any progress with his health. He has spent the entire time I've known him looking for a place to live. He has public housing assistance, but he has not been able to find anything suitable for a chemically sensitive person. He still has no place to live.

Eleanor called me for the first time about a health problem she was having and she continued to call regularly after that. She was a housewife, who had always been a little sensitive. In the spring, she had trouble with seasonal allergies. Also, at times, chemicals bothered her. However, she had been able to live a normal, happy life with her husband and son. Her serious health problems began when she had a new kitchen installed. Within a year of the installation, she developed serious symptoms. She became very chemically sensitive.

Eleanor believed that if only she could correct her house, she would get well. So, she had another kitchen put in. This time she tried to use all the correct materials; however, her health didn't improve.

Still, she made changes in her home, and each time she got a little worse. She could not seem to understand how MCS occurred or how to manage her life.

Eleanor became confined to her bedroom and, at this point, had become allergic to foods, pollens, and chemicals. It was going to be quite a challenge for her to recover!

When I first conversed with her, she had many doubts about energy healing and other alternative treatment methods. Being very analytical and skeptical about healing, she constantly questioned how various techniques worked.

However, gradually Eleanor changed. She began to believe in the power of the mind and positive thinking, and their influences on healing. Eventually, she grew more open to energetic healing techniques and began to explore new methods.

One of her new healing modalities was music. Eleanor loved music and found it helped her to release emotions. She grew stronger and stronger as she listened to various selections of music. She even listened to my cassette for enjoyment!

I admired Eleanor, for she was a very brave and determined woman; she was relentless about finding an answer. Her attention was focused on learning about different healing alternatives. Much of her time was devoted to calling others who were improving and inquiring about the healing method being employed. Even when she experienced setbacks, she held on tenaciously to the hope that someday she would eventually recover and enjoy life again.

Kathy was a teacher who had been exposed to roofing fumes a year after I had been. We discussed the exact same gut-wrenching pain in the right side of our bodies the night after the exposure at school. Our guess was that it might have been an injury to our livers. After that, we had become sensitive. The right side of her brain had also been affected, again as had mine. We had so many similar problems. We shared this bond.

Kathy had also been a musician. She had a beautiful speaking voice and I guessed that she must have been a wonderful singer. As was the case with me, she couldn't play her instruments (the violin and mandolin) for her ears had also been affected.

The only difference was that Kathy expressed her anger. She directed her outrage at the school and the chemicals. She fought relentlessly and won all her benefits. It helped me to hear her anger, for I was mostly heartbroken. I blamed myself for not being able to withstand the fumes. I also admonished myself for staying in the building, even after I knew the fumes were bothering me. In a way, Kathy's anger was good for me to hear. She was very supportive and encouraged me to stand up for my rights.

Kathy was instrumental in helping me to release the sentiments I felt but had not been able to express. Prior to our conversations, my reaction to the injury was a numb sense of shock. I was still trying to grasp that it had really happened. Kathy snapped me out of the fog of disbelief. It was not healthy for me to live in self-blame and distress. After discussions with Kathy, I was able to feel disgust at the poor judgment used in forcing me to breathe harmful substances while I was attempting, in good faith, to contribute to the educational process. I was needlessly injured and I had a right to be angry. It felt good inside to express my feelings and to allow for the release of the indignation.

Later, Kathy realized that eventually the anger has to end and her energy needed to be focused on her healing. Perhaps I helped her to see that constant anger was not healthy either; it can become destructive. She gradually accepted the fact that she would have to allow her body to heal; it was time to move on. I reminded her that we only have today— we must make the most of it. We must deal with what we have been handed; dwelling on anger and regrets only makes us, and those around us, miserable.

It seemed that I guided her out of her fury and she helped me express my lacking emotions. We acted as a balance for each other. My gratitude to Kathy is deep and I was very lucky to have known her through the difficult years following my injury.

Jenny deserves special mention, for she remained my friend and she was well! She had been my friend at school for years. When I was injured, she was teaching at another school. She didn't quite understand what was going on with me, but still she called. During the first year our friendship was very strained. I found it difficult to listen to her stories of the fun she was having with all of our friends. I sat alone day after day while she was still "living." I didn't understand why this had happened to me.

She found it difficult to understand MCS. I could hear the doubt in her voice. She would tell me to stop researching and trying to find answers. She thought I should just ignore the symptoms and carry on. If only I could have!

One day while we were talking, Jenny told me she had had a low blood sugar problem in the store. She had begun to shake and feel terrible. She said that she had run out of the store and hurried home to eat. I agreed with her that she had done the right thing but then, I asked her why she hadn't just ignored the symptoms and stayed in the store! Now she could see what it might be like to feel that way all the time, anywhere she went. It was just not possible for me to ignore the symptoms.

A year into my illness, her town began having difficulties in one of its schools. Teachers and students were becoming ill from the poor air quality and mysterious fumes. She read about this in the paper and started to believe in me more. Our friendship became more stable. She kept me informed of all the goings on at the school and I adjusted to hearing them. I needed to be connected to the outside world, even if it was painful. She was a wonderful friend. I look forward to seeing her again someday.

These are the dear people who kept me company during those years of isolation. Tenderly and lovingly, they reached across the miles to hold my hand and give me solace. In return I was able to comfort them in their time of need. We shared our dismal plights and knew we were not alone anymore. These friends were generous gifts from God. I continue to speak with all of them, and they have filled my heart with a special kind of love I will never forget.

Although my memory recalls many of the wonderful talks we enjoyed, there was one phone conversation that stood out among all the rest. . . .

Chapter 8

LORRI—DON'T DIE!

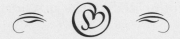

O ne evening in March, I received an unusual phone call. Generally, I heard from no one, except my MCS friends. The sicker I became, the less I heard from the outside world. David and my mother tried to convince relatives and friends to call me to keep me company, but very few did.

Ping only communicated with me once during my illness, but it was a communication that I shall never forget. She lived across the street from me. She was a friendly, direct Asian lady. She called and we talked for awhile. Since coming to the United States, she, too, had become sensitive. She said that she understood what I was going through. A while back, she also had endured a serious health problem with her thyroid.

Before she hung up, her last words of encouragement were words I held onto for the duration of my illness. She paused when we were about to say goodbye, and emphatically said, *"Lorri . . . don't die!"*

PART II

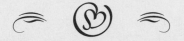

The way is not around, but rather over the obstacle. God is speaking and I am listening. I must prepare the new path to transcend the obstacle. I am weak and tired, and the work is hard. The Blessed Mother assists me and keeps me safe.

Chapter 9

FINDING THE ANSWER

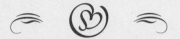

*B*y March of 1996, I was desperately clinging onto my life. My illness had lasted now for a year and a half. I was sliding downward constantly. I kept becoming allergic to more and more of the substances around me. Life was unbearable. Alone every day, I sat in my chair. Three or four phone calls a day from my friends sustained me. There was nothing else I could do.

I was seeing many doctors. They included my initial internist in Boston and the very caring doctor in Newburyport, Dr. Kinderlehrer. I had also continued to see the doctor in Connecticut, Dr. Green. He used homeopathy and Chinese herbs, but for some reason they weren't helping. My health continued to deteriorate. One evening, I looked woefully at him and said, "You keep trying to heal my body, but what about my mind?"

He looked helplessly at me. I finally had to admit that this treatment was not working. I wasn't sure where else to turn, but I knew that I needed to do something about my distressed mental state; I just couldn't take any more suffering. I was extremely frightened about what was happening to my body.

David had bought me a very large book for my birthday. It was entitled, *Alternative Medicine,* compiled by the Burton Goldberg Group. In it many types of healing methods were described. Phone numbers were listed at the conclusion of each section.

I asked David to look up hypnotherapy. Having majored in psychology as an undergraduate, I had always been interested in the mind and how it affects our health. Now I needed to find a way to control and direct my mind toward healing. I could no longer bear the fear and confusion in which I was living.

David read to me the section on hypnotherapy, and he wrote down the phone number at the end of the chapter. I called the next day and received a list of hypnotherapists in my area. I contacted a woman in my town and arranged to meet her at her home. Perhaps if I could reach my subconscious mind, I could help my ailing body.

I was easily hypnotized, but she said many negative things that seemed to make me uneasy. She did not understand about EI. One of her suggestions was to "kill all the bad cells in my body." When you are "under" and in a deep hypnotic state and you hear the word "kill," it can be very upsetting. Besides, I wasn't sure that I would have many good cells left if I killed off all the bad ones! She seemed very gentle, but I kept feeling tense during the session due to the disturbing suggestions.

Although I was a novice in the field of hypnosis, an inner awareness warned me about dealing with such an important part of the mind in a careless way. My mind needed reassurance and strength—not destruction within my body as suggested by this therapist. Who could I trust with this delicate task?

I looked for another way to benefit from hypnosis. This time I ordered a tape about general healing. Each night I listened to it. My health declined during that week. Now I realize that the suggestions in this tape were also inappropriate. It kept mentioning eating less and losing weight, and I was already thirty pounds underweight. I needed to eat more and gain weight! I realized that I needed to learn hypnosis myself so that I could make suggestions that were appropriate for me.

I called another number in the back of the book. It was a school where a person could study hypnotherapy, known as The American Institute of Hypnotherapy (AIH) in Irvine, California. I called and spoke to a doctor there. He talked to me about the mind and healing. He explained the doctoral program they offered as a distance learning program. It sounded very interesting.

Perhaps in this way, I could truly learn how to use hypnosis effectively. Also, I could be accomplishing something positive during this very dismal time of my life. My attention could be focused on something new and interesting. This was a wonderful and promising prospect for me. A tiny sensation of hope was felt within for the first time in years. However, the stronger feelings of doubt and fear rose up to quell it. How could I accomplish the requirements without the ability to read a book, or even hold a pen in my hand to write? There had to be a way!

That evening I talked to David about the doctoral program. David was interested but wondered how I would do this considering my limitations. Still, I was interested. I knew if I could learn hypnosis, I could reach a deep level of relaxation to assist my mind and learn what I needed in order to recover.

I called AIH the next day and spoke to the very polite admissions director. When I informed him that I couldn't read books, he suggested books on tape. This was a great idea. I was getting excited. I could have a purpose and a goal in life!

I signed up for the program and arranged for the tape recorder. But when it arrived, much to my dismay, I was unable to tolerate the recorder—it was new plastic and I could not have anything plastic in the room. Making matters worse, the sound was too difficult for my ears. I was discouraged. How could I read?

Then I got a bright idea. If I got a glass lasagna dish, I could put it over the book and read through it, without breathing any fumes. So, I ordered a lasagna dish and my first books from AIH.

My excitement was growing as I waited each day for the arrival of my items. The dish was delivered first and then I received my books. The first book I read was, *Getting Well Again,* by Carl and Stephanie Matthews Simonton. They worked with cancer patients. Their findings were very interesting and I began to see that our beliefs and our mind *can* change the course of an illness. They wrote:

> It is our central premise that an illness is not purely a physical problem, but rather a problem of the whole person, that it includes not only body but mind and emotions. We believe that emotional and mental states play a significant role both in susceptibility to disease, including cancer, and in recovery from all disease.[1]

They also wrote about biofeedback. This science teaches people to control a wide range of internal physical states, normally considered to be under involuntary control by the autonomic nervous system.

The Simontons discussed Elmer and Alyce Green of the Menninger Clinic, who were pioneers in the field of biofeedback. They believed that there was a very close connection between the physiological state and the mental/emotional state on both the conscious and unconscious levels. In their words, "The

---

[1] **Chapter 9:** Carl O. Simonton and Stephanie Matthew's Simonton, *Getting Well Again* (New York, NY: Bantam Books, 1992), 10.

mind, body, and emotions are a unitary system—affect one and you affect the others."[2]

Also Dr. Barbara Brown, another expert in biofeedback, stated, "Biofeedback is the first medically testable indication that the mind can relieve illnesses as well as create them."[3]

As I read this first book, I began to see that I needed to become aware of my own role in my illness. I could choose to live in the illness, or I could choose to control my mind and heal it.

I read on as the Simontons described using relaxation, imagery, exercise, and diet to enhance the body's natural immune defense system. My new course was set. I would learn all I could to help myself, for no one else could change the course of this illness.

I learned about the history of hypnosis. I found it interesting that hypnosis had been long used to assist in the healing process.

I was surprised to discover that hypnosis had been used during Egyptian times. There were "sleep temples" where priests put worshipers to "sleep" and made suggestions that they get well—and they usually did! These temples continued into Roman times.

Later, in the first century, the English Church supported the practice of "laying on of hands" as a healing technique. It was encouraged and perfected by the English monarch, Edward the Confessor, (1042–1066 A.D.) who was famous for his "royal touch."

As the British royalty eventually lost interest in the notion of "suggestion-healing," it fell into disrepute.

The power of suggestion was again introduced in France by Franz Anton Mesmer in the late 1700s. His practice was called "mesmerism" and "animal magnetism." This technique became popular with

---

[2] Ibid. p. 31.
[3] Ibid. p. 31.

the French nobility. It is reported that as many as three thousand people a day sought Mesmer's touch.[4]

His dramatic method involved having a group of people immerse themselves in a tub, or *baquet,* filled with water and iron filings. A magnetic influence was sought by holding on to iron rods. Mesmer would appear in his elegant silk robe, and his "animal magnetism" would be exuded. After going into convulsions, the patients would be taken into the recovery room to return to a normal state, and hopefully be healed.[5]

Under the direction of the King of France, a group of envious physicians and politicians, including Benjamin Franklin, joined together and investigated Mesmer. His flamboyant personality disturbed these austere men. They concluded that the healing effects Mesmer achieved were resulting from imagination and not from the iron rods. This finding discredited and disgraced Mesmer. Consequently, he was placed in exile. At that time, the idea of suggestion and imagination was not yet considered important.

The first physician to use hypnosis seriously was James Braid (1795–1860). He introduced the terms "hypnosis" and "hypnotist" and "suggestion." The word "hypnosis" derives from the Greek word *hypnos,* which means sleep. Braid realized that the word was misleading, since the person being hypnotized remains awake and actually very focused. However, by the time he realized this, it was too late to change the term; "hypnosis" had already caught on.

Dr. James Esdaile (1818–1859) was a personal friend of James Braid. While serving in India, he experimented with hypnosis as an anesthetic, which re-

---

[4] A. M. Krasner, Ph.D. *The Wizard Within* (Santa Anna, CA: American Board of Hypnotherapy Press, 1991), 11–13.

[5] Ernest R. Hilgard and Josephine R. Hilgard, *Hypnosis in the Relief of Pain* (New York, NY: Brunner/Mazel, 1994).

sulted in a reduction of the mortality rate during surgery to less than 5 percent. He experienced outstanding success. When he returned to England, Esdaile thought that his success would continue, but it didn't. Perhaps it was due to a difference in attitude. Indian culture embraces the concept of a "higher self," and spiritual practices such as meditation and altered states. This type of culture may benefit greatly from hypnosis, whereas a society that is closed to these ideas, such as England, may not. Thus, Esdaile failed in England. He lived the rest of his life in humiliation.

Late in the 1800s, Freud used hypnosis for a short time. He then abandoned it and used psychoanalysis. However, his method of free association may indeed have tapped into the subconscious mind and been a form of hypnosis.

I found one man especially interesting. He was a French pharmacist who worked in the early 1900s named Emile Coué. He taught the power of self-hypnosis, and in particular, "waking suggestion." His well-known expression was, "Every day in every way, I am getting better and better." This became my favorite saying throughout my healing. If things were going wrong and I felt scared, I would repeat this phrase. At first I didn't believe it, but I kept saying it. Soon, as I began to improve, the words rang truer and truer.

Coué also explained that if you hurt a part of your body, you should sit quietly and wave a hand over the affected area and say very quickly, "It is going. It is going." Saying the sentences quickly together allows no thought to come between the sentences. Thus, if we actually think it is going, it becomes a reality.[6]

---

[6] A. M. Krasner, Ph.D. *The Wizard Within,* (Santa Anna, CA: American Board of Hypnotherapy Press, 1991), 13–17.

Coué also advised:

> When you wish to do something reasonable, or when you have a duty to perform, always think it is easy. Make the words 'difficult' and 'I cannot' disappear from your vocabulary. Tell yourself, 'I can, I will, I must!'[7]

With my new knowledge growing and my belief that I, indeed, had a role in healing my own illness, I began to work with self-hypnosis. I was only a novice, but I was beginning to get the idea. At least I was being very careful about what I was thinking and saying to myself. As Emmett E. Miller wrote in his book *Deep Healing,*

> Our self-talk is a powerful inner mechanism through which we can make dramatic changes in our lives. It can affect every part of our being—mental, emotional, physical, and spiritual. As such, I consider this kind of inner talk to be one of the key tools we need to develop for deep healing.[8]

Along with my inner words and thoughts, I began to pay attention to the images I was forming in my mind. I realized that picturing my own funeral was certainly not the right idea if I wished to live, and I did. Instead, I had to picture myself well and happy. I needed to send a clear positive message to my inner self. I wanted to heal!

Finally, after a year and a half, I was on my way. Realizing that I played a major part in my own recovery, I began to feel a little optimistic. Gradually, my own power was emerging and I was preparing for the role of a lifetime—healing myself! The way was opening up and it was time to venture into this new territory.

---

[7] Ibid. p. 194.

[8] Emmett E. Miller, M.D. *Deep Healing: The Essence of Mind/Body Medicine* (Carlsbad, CA: Hay House Inc. 1997), 103–104.

Chapter 10

MY PRAYER IS HEARD

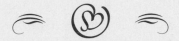

*I*t was the last week in April—three weeks since I had begun reading my hypnosis assignments under the lasagna dish. I was still having great difficulty living my daily life. My entire wardrobe consisted of the one dreary outfit—my husband's gray sweatshirt and my gray corduroys. I worried all the time about becoming allergic to them. What then would I do?

I remained in one room and couldn't go out in the daylight. Even indoors, I was wearing sunglasses. Light was extremely painful for me. Sound, too, was difficult, so I lived in my quiet world, alone and frightened.

One day I received a call from a woman in Vermont. She had bought my Christian tape, recorded two years prior to my illness. I had written some of the songs and had received a *Billboard* music certificate for one of them. The tapes were still in circulation. One song was written by a healing priest named, Father McDonough. The song was called "Gentle Shepherd." It was the only song Father wrote, and he said it had just come to him. It was very beautiful.

This woman called to tell me how much she had loved the music. I was very touched. When she asked me where I sang, I had to tell her that I was very ill. She listened to me very quietly. Then she asked me if I had gone to Father McDonough for a healing. I had not. I explained that I had been too ill to go to one of his services. She encouraged me to call his prayer line.

Her advice touched me deeply, and after we hung up, I dialed the prayer line. Father wasn't there, but I spoke to an assistant. I told her in a very shaky voice about my plight. I asked her to pray for me. We prayed together.

The next day, a wonderful thing happened. I called a company in Oregon from which I ordered herbs. While speaking with a doctor there, I asked for advice about my cotton allergy. I told him how I could not wear clothes. He listened and then he said the nicest words I think I have ever heard. They were, "You know, there is a cure for allergies." I thought I was dreaming. I asked if I had heard him correctly, He elaborated and explained that allergies can be cleared by the body and the result is permanent. I was astonished. I had prayed and prayed for this. I was so afraid that I would have to live my entire life suffering and unable to wear clothes.

He gave me the phone number in California to call, which I did immediately. It was the number of Dr. Devi Nambudripad who had invented a treatment called the Nambudripad Allergy Elimination Technique (NAET™). The lovely lady who answered was Dr. Nambudripad's sister, Mala. When I explained where I was from, she informed me that there was a doctor in my state who had studied with Dr. Nambudripad and had learned her treatment. He was only forty minutes away! The amazing thing was that I had spoken with his partner, Patricia Hughes, just three days before. She had told me something about this treatment, but I had not grasped what she meant, because she had used a term that I did not understand—"energetic clearing" and it did not register. I guess God needed to drill this point home by having the doctor in Oregon tell me about it yet again!

Thank goodness he did, for I called Dr. Robert Sampson and Patricia Hughes and made an appointment for the next day.

David drove. I was still wearing a blindfold and sat in the back seat so as to be protected from the light. David and I joked that if we were stopped, he would have a lot of explaining to do to convince the policeman that he wasn't kidnapping me. I sure looked strange.

When we arrived at the house they used for treating patients, I met Dr. Sampson and Patricia Hughes. They were caring and warm. Sitting in front of him in my tattered gray outfit, I told Dr. Sampson of my difficulty wearing clothes. As he listened kindly, I explained all my problems. He related to me that Patricia had also become unable to tolerate her own clothes, because she had treated them with ozone to eliminate paint fumes from them. She found that she was unable to tolerate the ozone odor on the clothes. As a result of this, she was left with nothing of her own to wear. Consequently, she had had to use his clothes. He went on to recount his own difficulties with Environmental Illness. He explained that they had both been ill for years and were well now. I knew that I was in the right place and that they understood!

Dr. Sampson began to "balance" me. I had no idea what was going on. He kept asking my body questions and pushing down on my arm. He made strange arm movements and had me make them as well. Then he made a strange noise to adjust my chakra. I was bewildered. My very patient husband watched and did not know what to think.

Dr. Sampson was using an advanced balancing treatment devised by Stephen Rochlitz. Rochlitz is the author of the book, *Allergies and Candida: with the Physicist's Rapid Solution.*

In his text, Rochlitz relates his struggle to recover his health for many years. He tried many solutions and finally studied kinesiology. He writes about his breakthrough:

> Then I became aware of kinesiology (also called Touch for Health and muscle testing and balancing). At a seminar in 1983, I learned of a previously developed method of 'asking the body questions' or balancing the body's energies for a specific problem. The brain records everything that has happened to it and the muscle testing is just a biofeedback system to get at this knowledge.[1]

Also in his book, Rochlitz explains the development of kinesiology. He relates that, in the early 1960s, a man named George Goodheart, D.C. (doctor of chiropractic) discovered that testing minute changes in muscle strength could provide a useful feedback system. Goodheart expanded on the basic knowledge of kinesiology (which had already existed), when he realized that there was an energetic connection between the individual muscles and the body's acupuncture meridian system. The meridian

---

system consists of pathways of energy conducted throughout the body, bringing energy to the organs. This indicates that a feedback system exists between the muscles, acupuncture meridians, and the organs. By testing muscle strength, the condition of the correlating acupuncture meridian can be determined and the energy of the organ can be measured.

Goodheart named his work, "Applied Kinesiology," and this knowledge was shared within the chiropractic community.

According to Rochlitz, "Applied Kinesiology can gauge imbalance and help restore balance to muscles, meridians, spine, lymph, and circulatory systems."[2]

This was what Dr. Sampson was working with. He kept asking my body questions, sometimes even silently! I kept responding, as my muscle tested "weak" or "strong." Based on my answer, he would make a move or change in my body. Then, he would retest and voilà, the muscle test would change. I had absolutely no idea what he was doing, but I was so sick that I just stood there and let him work.

Then it was time for my Nambudripad treatment. Again, Dr. Sampson used kinesiology to muscle test me. He had me hold a tiny vial with a potential allergen in it and he pushed on my arm. If it went weak, I was sensitive to the substance in the vial.

Dr. Nambudripad has designed a protocol that must be carefully followed. She has determined that there are some basic elements that must be cleared before others may be addressed. Some of the necessary items to clear first are substances such as sugar, salt, vitamin A, the B vitamins, vitamin C, minerals, eggs, and chicken. It is her contention that the body

_____

[2] Ibid. pp. 105-107.

is able to be strengthened by these preliminary treatments. Consequently, treatments of other allergens will clear more easily and with greater success.

Muscle testing revealed that I was "weak" for sugar—this was to be my first treatment.

After Robert cleared my energy meridians, it was time for Patricia to come into the room and massage the "gate points"—specific acupuncture points on the hands, arms, and feet that open the energy meridians. When she entered the room, I felt as if my own angel of healing had come in. Her gentle presence felt wonderful. She reassured me and spoke of healing. My prayers were being answered and I was going to be well. Patricia talked about how the Blessed Mother had played a role in her healing. I was surprised to hear this. I then confided in Patricia how the Blessed Mother had also guided me. And now I believed that perhaps the Blessed Mother had lovingly directed me to Patricia and Robert.

That evening I felt completely relaxed and wonderful. Something had changed in me and I was relieved. Now, with my use of hypnosis and this new therapy, perhaps there would be a life after MCS. . . .

Chapter 11

DR. DEVI NAMBUDRIPAD

*I*n early May of 1996, my study of hypnosis was
progressing slowly—but it was progressing.
Reading through the lasagna dish was tiring for
my eyes, but I persisted for as long as possible each
day. Completing the papers was impossible, due to
my inability to write with a pen or use a computer.
David had suggested that I dictate my findings to
him, so he could type them on the computer. We accomplished a little of this task once in awhile, but he
seemed so tired in the evenings that I didn't feel
right asking him to work more for me. Each paper
was required to be minimum of twenty pages and
there were twenty-eight papers! This would take a
long time at the rate we were going! However, my determination was strong and I secretly decided that I
would only require assistance for the first ten papers—by then I would have healed enough to write
and type my own. Along with my hypnosis work with
AIH, I was learning more and more about the amazing contribution of Dr. Devi Nambudripad. Her remarkable discovery of how to eliminate allergies had

me intrigued. I ordered her book from California and eagerly awaited its arrival.

That week, I received Dr. Nambudripad's book called, *Say Good-By To Illness.* Dr. Nambudripad was an acupuncturist when she first realized how to eliminate allergies. One day she began having a reaction to carrots she had just eaten. Attempting an acupuncture treatment on herself to reduce the reaction, she discovered that she had done more than relieve the problem. She had eliminated the allergy completely; she no longer reacted to carrots. Dr. Nambudripad wondered what was different about this particular treatment. She remembered that she still had some pieces of carrot near her while she performed the treatment. The idea came to her that by having the energy of the substance present while she cleared the meridians, she had somehow altered her pattern of response to the carrot.

Dr. Nambudripad, who had been very ill with Multiple Chemical Sensitivities and food allergies, able to eat only broccoli and rice, had been living a very difficult life. This new discovery changed all that. Eventually it would also improve the lives of so many others! Dr. Nambudripad also realized that:

> Through 31 pairs of spinal nerves, the brain operates the largest network of communication within the body. Energy blockages happen in a person's body due to contact with adverse energy of other substances. When two adverse energies come closer, repulsion takes place. When two similar energies get together, attraction takes place. The repulsion of energies is referred to in this book as an allergy. The repulsion of energies can happen between two living organisms, (e.g. between two humans, such as father and son; two siblings, husband and wife; two friends, animals and human being, etc.) It can also occur between one living organism and one non-living organ-

ism, for example, between a human being and fabrics or food . . . [1]

When we come in contact with another energy field to which we are allergic, our energy pathways become blocked. As a result of this contact, an organ manifests an allergic response. This is what allopathic doctors look at and treat—the obvious response. However, Dr. Nambudripad revealed another step occurring before the obvious reaction.

She began to develop a technique and to perfect it. She realized from working with people that allergies can be at the root of many illnesses. Usually we associate allergies with asthma, rashes, hives, sneezing, or coughing. She saw that "There is hardly a human disease or condition that may not involve an allergic factor."[2] Illnesses such as chronic fatigue, fibromyalgia, arthritis, and other problems in the body can also have allergies as their root cause. Clear the allergies and resolve the illness. Dr. Nambudripad also understood that:

> There is no limit to the number and kinds of substances that cause allergic reactions. Any substance under the sun, including sunlight, can cause an allergic reaction in any individual. In our highly technological age, the number of substances that are potentially allergenic are constantly being expanded as we learn what it truly means to 'live better through chemistry.'[3]

One possible explanation that Dr. Nambudripad offers for the development of sensitivities is that

---

[1] Devi S. Nambudripad, D.C., L.Ac., R.N., Ph.D. *Say Goodbye to Illness* (Buena Park, CA: Delta Publications, 1993), 9.

[2] Ibid. p. 3.

[3] Ibid. p. 6.

changes in the sensory nerve fibers of certain organs render them unable to conduct messages to and from the spinal cord and the brain. In some people, these dormant receptors result in *hyposensitivity* to certain items, while in others, they may result in *hypersensitivity*.

The *hypersensitive* group experiences obvious allergic reactions. The *hyposensitive* group experiences few blatant reactions, but may deal with poor health and inadequate function of the body and mind.

Hypersensitivity is called "active allergies." Whereas, *hyposensitivity* is called "hidden allergies."

Sometimes allergic conditions can be inherited. Depending on one's genetic predisposition, the age of onset may vary. In some people, the sensory nerve fibers become altered during their lifetime when they experience an event such as a major illness, an exposure to toxins, a severe reaction to drugs, chemicals, etc. When this occurs, injury to the sensory nerve fibers results, interfering with their conductivity.

Dr. Nambudripad has developed a technique that restores normal function to these sensory nerve fibers, which, in turn, restores normal function to the body parts or organs that these sensory nerve fibers supply.[4]

Since 1983, she has been working on her technique. It is now known as Nambudripad Allergy Elimination Technique (NAET™).

The principle of NAET™ is to first test the client and see if his/her muscles become weak when a substance is held. If so, it indicates that an allergy or sensitivity exists. Then certain acupuncture points are massaged on the back; after which, gate points are also massaged on the hands, arms, and feet. All

---

[4] Ibid. p. 5.

this is done while the person is holding onto the vial containing the allergenic substance. This process opens the energy meridians so that the body will learn that it does not need to shut down when in contact with the substance.

For the next twenty-five hours, the client should avoid contact with the substance so as not to interfere with the clearing. It takes two hours to clear each major meridian; there are twelve meridians. One extra hour is allotted to be sure the process has been completed.

After this time period, the person is retested. If the allergy has not yet cleared, another treatment is necessary. The muscle should test strong. It is also important to ask, using kinesiology, if it is *100 percent* clear. This is helpful, because at times the arm may test strong when the substance has cleared only 80 percent or more. The person may continue to react even though the arm tested strong. He/she may then think that the treatment did not process or that this method of allergy elimination doesn't work. Always make certain that it has cleared *100 percent*. It is a wonderful answer to a previously challenging situation.

Before, when a person developed allergies, the advice was always "avoidance." But how many things must we go around avoiding? *Life can become very difficult when we must avoid everything!* Also, as Nambudripad says:

> When such a person is surrounded by numerous adverse energies all the time, his/her energy pathways remain blocked all the time. The continuous blockage of the energy pathways causes poor body function.[5]

---

[5] Ibid. p. 10.

Once the energy meridians are opened for a certain substance, the body can benefit from it rather than become ill from it. For example, if a person is allergic to a mineral such as zinc, he may feel ill when he eats a meal high in zinc or attempts to take a supplement with zinc in it.

Also, as a result of the energy blockage existing within the body, the zinc may not be absorbed well into the system. This may occur because the energy blockage also serves to protect the person from absorbing the allergenic nutrient deep into the body. Often a deficiency can develop. After the treatment for zinc is completely cleared, zinc can once again be easily tolerated and assimilated into the body, thus strengthening the person. Dr. Nambudripad even suggests that a supplement be taken to build up the zinc levels.

Other nutrients, as well, contained within the food may not be utilized properly by the body when allergies are present. A person might become frustrated trying to take supplements, only to react to them and not benefit from them. Even if a person were trying to eat a nutritious diet, he may have been discouraged at his poor and weakened state. As more and more nutrients are gradually cleared, the body gains the benefits from these substances. Deficiencies that may have developed are resolved. After successful treatments, when the allergies are completely eliminated, the body may once again reap the benefits of a nutritious diet.

This is a wonderful treatment! Dr. Nambudripad offers people a chance at a new life. She has now trained many doctors throughout the country. Slowly, people are realizing that allergies can actually be eliminated—that our body's energy can be opened and our health restored!

Chapter 12

ANOTHER HURDLE

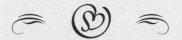

*A*fter my first meeting with Doctor Sampson, I was becoming hopeful. However, another problem began developing. I confided in David that I was experiencing dizzy spells, which were progressively getting worse.

One evening, when he was watching me read through the lasagna dish, he noticed how thick and wavy the glass was. He came over and tried to read through it. He couldn't believe that I had actually been spending hours reading this way. He said it made him dizzy in just minutes. He was certain that this was not a good idea and strongly suggested that I stop reading this way.

I felt that a huge door had been slammed in my face. How could I stop now? I had just gotten my books back after being without them for a year and a half.

I kept thinking of the movie *Farenheit 451,* which I had seen many years ago. It was a futuristic film wherein the government would burn any books it found. Some of the people dedicated their time to preserving books. By memorizing the books and reciting them aloud to each other, they kept the stories alive. It was such a struggle to keep their books. I felt that I was reliving this movie. I had always loved to read and now was being forced to live without my books. I felt lost.

For the next week, I sat at my dining room table (which was at the far end of my kitchen-dining room). Again, I sat all day in a chair and could do nothing but listen to the clock tick.

One day, as I sat at the table trying to figure out how to read, I thought about purchasing a "reading box." I had seen them in catalogs. They were boxes made of glass and some type of metal, constructed large enough to fit over a book. There was some kind of fan mechanism attached to the back to help direct fumes out the window. These boxes were extremely expensive, but I was desperate to figure out how to read so that I could heal myself. Suddenly, as I looked down at my table, a novel idea came to me. The dining room table was glass and had a wood frame all around it. Would it be possible to place a book under it somehow and read through the table? Perhaps.

I went over to the breakfast bar and picked up a little stool. I put it under the table. Then I got one of my books and placed it on the stool, under the table. Voilà! There I had it! I could read through the table and clearly see the book below. The glass was thin enough and not at all wavy. I was on my way again!

That night I showed David and asked him if he thought it would be all right to read through the table. He seemed amused. He thought it was fine. My spirits were lifted.

The only drawback that I experienced was a very painful neck and shoulders, which already hurt me from the injury. I decided to go to the chiropractor Dr. Deborah Miller every week, in order to relieve my aching neck and shoulders. When I told her how I was reading, she looked at me in amazement. At first, she must have thought I was crazy to bring myself such pain, but as time went on, she noticed the improvement in my health and my spirits. So, she attended to me, sustaining me through the "reading through the table" stage.

I was reading again and loving it!

Chapter 13

WHAT ARE YOU DOING?

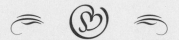

The last week in May, I went for my final visit to the doctor in Connecticut. I had not done well with him, but until now I had no other alternative. He tested me and seemed disturbed. He shook his head. He was puzzled. He looked up at me and asked me, "What are you doing, anyway? Everything has shifted." He was worried. I was elated! I kept hearing the words. "Everything has shifted!" Finally! That is what I needed.

He was concerned and gave me remedies to bring me back to the way I had been. I bought them, but upon careful consideration, I decided that I didn't want to go back to the way I had been. So, I left my body alone and let the shift happen.

I never returned to that doctor and decided, instead, to work with Robert Sampson and Patricia Hughes.

The next week, I returned to them for another treatment. I was looking forward to my appointment. I was feeling a little better for the first time in years. They were giving me so much hope.

Dr. Sampson began his complicated muscle testing. He was asking questions and having me make statements. I was getting interested in what was happening. I looked at him and asked, "What are you doing?" He explained that when he asked my body a question, if the arm went down easily when he pushed on my wrist, the answer was "yes." If it remained strong, it meant "no."

Then he further explained that when he made a statement, if the arm remained strong, it was "true." If the arm went weak, then the statement was "false."

I watched as he continued. This was the first thing Dr. Sampson taught me. Little did I know that he would open a whole new world for me and teach me so much more.

I was amazed that even when he asked the questions "silently" my body could still respond. What are the implications of this? Does this mean that we can "understand" what other people are thinking about us? Is that perhaps why we get an uneasy feeling around some people without knowing why? . . . perhaps we are feeling what they are thinking. It still gives me pause.

I went home that week and asked my husband to try the muscle testing. At first, we felt silly and could get nowhere. Each night we worked on it. After some practice, David became very proficient at getting answers for me. It made life so much easier to ask what I was reacting to. The answer was often correct and I could solve my problem.

If I could give one bit of advice to a person who is allergic to substances, it would be: learn how to muscle test. Have a friend or spouse try to assist you, and eventually learn to test yourself. The benefits are well worth it. Who would know better what you are reacting to than you yourself? It is a simple connection to your own subconscious.

How to Muscle Test

Here is a description of how to muscle test with the assistance of another person. (See Fig. 1.)

- First, stand and look straight ahead.
- Extend your arm directly out in front of you with your palm facing down. You can use either arm, but let's say you use your left arm.
- The person who will be testing stands on your right.
- He also extends his arm directly in front of him until his hand touches your wrist. He only needs to use three fingers to push down on your wrist.
- He should use his right arm since you are using your left. If he wishes, he can hold onto your right shoulder with his left hand for balance.
- Then hold the substance in question in your right hand.
- The tester pushes gently on your wrist. If your arm goes weak, then you might be sensitive to it. Try holding other objects in your hand as well to see the difference between strong and weak responses.
- Between each object you test, it is important that you rub your hands together a few times to clear the energy of the first substance from your hands. Then you are ready to test another substance. Muscle testing takes practice. At first,

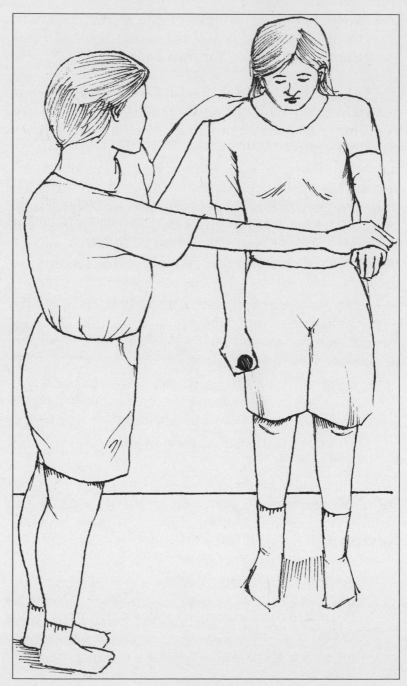

Fig. 1

you might feel uncomfortable. After you work on it, you can develop a reliable form of communication with your own body.

As I developed this skill with David's help, I eventually learned how to muscle test myself using my right index finger and pushing down with the left index finger. (See Fig. 2.) Instead of holding an item in my hand, I began asking questions about my reactions. This takes practice in order to arrive at clear answers that are not influenced by your conscious mind. It took me a long time to perfect this method, but once I caught on, I had a wonderful tool to use. I needed to develop an independent testing technique, for David was not always around to assist me.

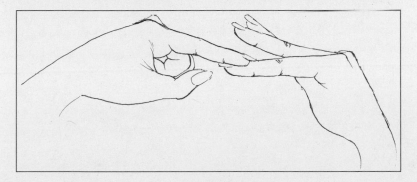

Fig. 2

Review

When asking a question:

- If the arm (or finger) feels **weak,** the answer is **"yes."**
- If the arm (or finger) remains **strong,** the answer is **"no."**

Begin by asking a question to which you already know the answer. One example might be, "Is my name _____?" Testing this will demonstrate the difference between a strong and weak response.

When issuing a statement:

- If the arm (or finger) remains **strong,** the statement is **true.**
- If the arm (or finger) feels **weak,** the statement is **false.**

Begin by stating a fact you can change to make true or false. One example might be, "My name is _____." This again will demonstrate the difference between a strong and weak response.

Chapter 14

TAPAS FLEMING

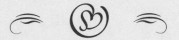

I t was late in May and I continued my appointments each week with Dr. Robert Sampson and Patricia Hughes. My body was extremely ill, but I was beginning to feel slight improvements. My weight had stabilized and my arms were not always weak and shaky. Hope was growing within. I continued to learn more techniques from Dr. Sampson. One very helpful and simple method was termed TAT™ (Tapas Acupressure Technique), named after its creator, Tapas Fleming.

TAT™ was discussed in Fleming's workbook called, *Reduce Traumatic Stress in Minutes*. In this manual, Tapas explains a technique she developed. She was an acupuncturist when she devised it. She, in fact, had been working with Dr. Devi Nambudripad at the time.

Robert encouraged me to order Tapas Fleming's book. There was a section about clearing past events as well as one for clearing allergies. Releasing traumas seemed like a positive step in healing, so I sent for the book.

Tapas states that traumatic experiences create energy blockages in the body, which remain with us long after the experience has gone away. She explains:

> A blockage or energy stagnation has just been put in place and your life has been impacted. . . . It is as if life were a flowing stream, and at one point, out of fear, you roll a boulder into it to try to dam the flow in order to keep a traumatic event from happening to you. The water, of course, simply flows around the boulder, but in your life—in your body, mind and emotions—there is a blockage that wasn't there before.[1]

She explains that the TAT™ (Tapas Acupressure Technique) can give you the opportunity to release this trauma and free up the blockage. According to Fleming:

> TAT™ is a way of saying to your whole body-mind, 'Have another look at this.' It is an opportunity to change, based on taking a new look, rather than continuing to look away. By taking another look, within the context of TAT's direction of the body's energy flow, the charge that is still being held is removed from the past event and the event can now be integrated into your whole system.[2]

If we have many traumatic events in our past, there can be many blockages. This can certainly be contributing to a state of poor health. I needed to do everything to help my body regain its energy flow and become vibrant again.

---

[1] **Chapter 14:** Tapas Fleming, L.Ac. *Reduce Traumatic Stress in Minutes* (TAT Workbook, 1996), 5.
[2] Ibid. p. 5.

I wasn't able to perform this energy work very often at home, because I was clearing allergies each week at my appointments with Dr. Sampson. Any energy shift is strongly felt when one is extremely sensitive. One energy session a week was adequate for me at this stage of healing. At times, when I took a break from my NAET™ treatments, I would clear a trauma. The method was so simple. Tapas explains the exact acupressure points on your head to touch and how to focus on the event. It only takes minutes.

I must caution that if you decide to work with this method, you should proceed slowly and carefully. Try clearing one trauma only and see how you feel just after and even into the next day. You can ask your body, by using muscle testing, how many traumas you can work on that day. I advise caution because each change is significant to a very sensitive person. Even though it seems simple, it is powerful and your body must process the adjustments after you do the treatment. Healing takes time and your body must integrate the information. Give it a chance and *be gentle*.

Chapter 15

JUST DON'T COME!

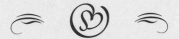

I t was June of 1996. I had seen Robert and Patricia for ten treatments so far. I was seeing slight improvements, but not nearly enough to feel healthy by the summer, which had always been my favorite time of year. This June a special event was approaching. I wanted to be ready for it, but I could not improve fast enough.

My younger brother was a superb athlete. We had been very close growing up. I had taken him to the tennis courts when he was very young, for I loved to play tennis. In the summer, I had played every night until the lights went out. When I had first brought my brother, he took to it immediately. Each night we had volleyed with our special group of friends, and my brother kept improving. He began winning small local tournaments. He loved the sport.

His talent extended to other sports as well. My older brother and I took him skiing and the same thing happened.

Later, in high school, he played basketball, baseball, and soccer. He was captain of all the teams. He won the title of "All State" at soccer. His natural athletic ability was clearly evident; he excelled at every sport he played.

I had enjoyed watching him develop into a superb athlete and it gave me much pride to see the little boy I had taken to the tennis courts grow into such a handsome and accomplished man. Now his day of recognition was upon us. He was being inducted into the local "Hall of Fame."

He contacted me first when he heard. He felt so honored that he had been selected. He called to see if there was any way I could attend. He urged me to try. While I was ill, he had been calling me each week long distance from his home in Connecticut. I knew he really could never imagine how sick I was. Sadly, I told him I didn't think it would be possible. This was very hard for me to say, for I so wanted to go.

During the week before the ceremony, everybody was getting excited. All my relatives were going. My brother's old friends from his high school teams were arriving from all areas of the country. It was all my family could talk about. One day, when I was talking with my mother, I hinted that maybe I could come to her house after the ceremony, where the people were gathering for a celebratory party. She immediately balked at the idea. She said. "What would you wear? You can't come in that!" She indicated my tattered gray sweatshirt and corduroys. I looked down at myself and saw that she was right. Then she continued. "And look at your hair. What can you do about that?" I touched my once beautiful long, highlighted, blond hair. Now it was dull brown and not very well styled, for I had to style it myself. It was not very pretty. She was right. She made it clear that it wasn't a good idea. Still, I wanted to come!

I even treated, using NAET™ with Dr. Sampson, for a nice pair of shorts and a tee shirt in the secret hope that I might somehow be able to go.

That weekend David had to go to a conference out of state. It was the first time he had dared to leave me alone since my injury. We were both nervous. I needed his help so much. We figured I would be all right with all my family around.

The night before the ceremony, my brother arrived from Connecticut. He called me that evening as he was preparing his speech. He wanted to see what I thought of it. I listened proudly. It was splendid. He did everything well. I gave some opinions. We talked. Everything was going well, until I said, "I'm going to try to come to Mom's after the ceremony." I then asked him if he could ask his friends' wives and girlfriends not to wear perfume so that I could be present.

Immediately, he responded. He said that it would be too difficult to reach them now. They were staying in all different places. He just couldn't do it. He then added that it would be too difficult to reach all our relatives as well. Then he said very matter-of-factly, "Just . . . don't come!"

Tears welled up in my eyes. "Just, don't come!" How easy it was for him to say. But, I wanted to come. I wanted to be part of my family's life. I was now always left out. I was sick of it.

I knew he was right, logically, but there comes a time when Environmental Illness becomes horrible and tiring. This night was one of those times. I realized that night that I had become an embarrassment and a burden to my family. They didn't seem to want to deal with me and all the trouble I created. It was just too inconvenient.

I felt terrible. When David called to tell me he had arrived safely at his destination, I cried to him over the phone. He felt so sorry, but there was nothing he could do for me.

My mother called; my brother and she must have discussed the possibility of my coming. She began to figure how they could reach everybody. I was upset and just said, "Never mind." I honestly knew it was too difficult. I didn't even have a ride—I couldn't drive myself and David was away. I couldn't handle the light if they sat outside, and I couldn't handle the fragrances if they sat inside. Just forget it!

I didn't sleep all night. My mother didn't either. She was so loving, but the illness was just too difficult to deal with.

The next day, the day of the ceremony, I sat in my chair, alone, listening to the clock tick. I watched the time drag on and on. Finally, I figured it was time for his speech. I sent him my love and wished him luck. I was so proud of him, but I felt I had failed him—I should have been there.

Weeks later, I watched the video of his award and his speech—he was wonderful. He mentioned all the people who had been there for him. I was not mentioned.

It was one of the sad times of my life. I vowed that I would not be left out again. I was even more determined to get well.

Chapter 16

HOPEFUL SUMMER

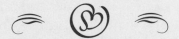

T he summer of 1996 I was feeling a bit stronger. It was a much more optimistic time.

I was still unable to go out in the light. However, something in me had improved and now I could be in the car for about one hour if I wore double sunglasses. This made me very happy.

Still, I spent every day inside until 6:30 P.M. This was an improvement over the previous summer. Back then, I couldn't go out until 7:30, when it had begun to get dark.

I decided to devote this summer to studying and using hypnosis. I had read a few books about healing with hypnosis, and the more I read, the more I was convinced that I could greatly direct my healing with the right hypnosis treatments.

One more hurdle remained to achieve my doctorate. I had to complete the twenty-eight papers. During this season, I was dictating the work to David. This was a difficult and slow process.

In order to facilitate the project, I asked Dr. Sampson to treat me, using NAET™, for a yellow pen, so that I could begin writing out the papers.

Writing each twenty/thirty-page paper by hand required a great deal of effort, but it was the best I could do at that time. After I completed each paper, David would type it out. This was a bit more convenient for both of us.

I kept in mind my secret plan of only letting David type out ten papers. By that point, I intended to be well enough to type the rest myself.

Now that I was able to write the papers, I had something to occupy my time during the interminably long days. Thank goodness for my studies.

As I studied hypnosis, I read the works of some very insightful authors. Their views on the power and effects of hypnosis were interesting and enlightening. One of my favorite books was written by the director of my school, Dr. Krasner. This excellent book was entitled, *The Wizard Within.* He wrote, "Your subconscious mind controls the health and function of every cell, of every organ, bone, tissue, etc. that is contained in your body."[1]

My work with Dr. Sampson and Patricia reinforced the concept that our state of health is directly related to our thoughts and emotions. Most of my friends with EI kept insisting that the condition was purely physical. I had thought this initially. It is a difficult realization that every thought and feeling can influence your illness. But in another light, if you are positive, you can direct yourself out of an illness.

Barbara Ann Brennan writes in her book, *Hands of Light:*

> Responsibility and acceptance promote power, power from within to create your reality. For if you uncon-

---

[1] **Chapter 16:** A. M. Krasner, *The Wizard Within* (Santa Anna, CA: American Board of Hypnotherapy Press, 1991), 76.

sciously had something to do with making things the way they are, then you can have a great deal to do with creating things the way you want them to be.[2]

As soon as I began to think in this manner, I realized that I had an important role in healing myself. I felt empowered rather than discouraged.

I now understand that any illness is not just physical. There is always a component of the mental and emotional contained within it. We are not simply these physical shells walking around. We are constantly feeling emotions and having thoughts about our life. These events, of course, affect us directly. In Dr. Krasner's words:

> Your life is the direct result of your previous and present thoughts, desires, and emotions. . . . If you take the trouble to watch your thoughts, literally notice what you are thinking every day, you will find that you automatically and undeliberately do a lot of negative "picturing" in your mind. These mental pictures set in motion the forces to cause these pictures to actually develop into reality. . . . 'Picture it and it shall be.'[3]

So, I was trying to be aware of what I was thinking—even when I was not specifically using hypnosis. Patricia taught me to try to notice exactly what I was thinking just prior to a reaction. Sometimes I saw that she was right. I would be thinking, "Oh boy, I'm going to have trouble with that," and then, guess what? I would react to the substance.

---

[2] Barbara Ann Brennan, *Hands of Light* (New York, NY: Bantam Books, 1988), 133.

[3] A. M. Krasner, *The Wizard Within* (Santa Anna, CA: American Board of Hypnotherapy Press, 1991), 176.

Other times, I really couldn't see a connection between my thoughts and the reaction. Still, I attempted to say only positive expressions and to ask others around me to please say positive remarks to me. At first it was strange, for we make so many negative statements. We limit ourselves constantly. People with EI often say, "I'll never go near that substance again." "I'll never be able to shop in that store again." "That scent is bad." We need to realize that many things in our environment aren't so detrimental. They are only difficult for us because they cause us to react. When the reaction is calmed, they can be wonderful for us once again.

This kind of understanding took a long time for me, with the constant coaching and assistance from Patricia. She taught me not to be afraid of the world that had seemed to have become my enemy.

That summer, I focused my attention on saying and thinking positive words. I continued to repeat my favorite expression of Emile Coué, "Every day in every way, I am getting better and better." I said this every day even when I really didn't believe it at the time. The more I said it, the more it became my reality. Dr. Krasner put it well when he said, "When we believe something or believe in something, we are delivering a message to the brain about what is occurring. The brain then orders the body how to respond."[4]

The more I read about the mind and healing, the more I was convinced that I had control over this injury. Perhaps it would take time, but I could do it—if I persevered.

As summer ended and fall began, I read my assignments from the American Institute of Hyp-

---

[4] Ibid. p. 3.

notherapy. One assignment was Deepak Chopra's book, *Quantum Healing*. Through many interesting examples, he explores the mind/body connection.

One story about his mother's allergy was quite interesting. He relates that his mother had a specific allergy to pollen which was found in Jammu, her home. One time when his mother was returning home on an airplane, she thought they were landing at Jammu right at peak season for the pollen to be out. She began reacting. The steward asked what was wrong. She explained that she always reacted to the pollen at Jammu. He was surprised and explained that they were not landing at Jammu, but were landing at another stop first.[5] How do we explain her sudden allergy? If her mind could elicit this reaction, could we be causing many or all of our own problems?

I remember a dramatic event in my own life that shows the power of the mind.

During the summer of 1973, my grandmother became very ill and was taken to the hospital. The doctor didn't know what was wrong with her. He had given her all kinds of tests.

My older brother was to be married the following week. Although my grandmother was very weak, she was still very excited about the wedding. She insisted on attending. She begged and begged until the doctor released her from the hospital. She seemed to come alive. The night before, she had her hair styled. My aunt bought her a pretty dress and she happily prepared for the event. The day of the wedding she smiled constantly. She laughed at jokes and enjoyed everybody. It was wonderful to see her have so much fun.

---

[5] Deepak Chopra, M.D. *Quantum Healing: Exploring the Frontiers of Mind/Body Medicine* (New York, NY: Bantam Books, 1989), 118.

That evening we all went to bed smiling. What a wonderful time we had had. The next morning, I received a call from my uncle. He told me that my grandmother had died in her sleep with a smile on her face.

How amazing that she stayed alive just long enough to attend her grandson's wedding! How wonderful to have spent the last day of her life happy and surrounded by all her loving family!

Deepak Chopra cites many experiences that are similar to this. He tells of a man who was in good health until he was informed that there was a tumor inside him. He had lived with this tumor for years without being aware of it. Three months after hearing about it, he was dead.[6] How does this happen? Is the mind that powerful?

According to Chopra, the *rishis* (ancient seers of India) gave much thought to the fundamental nature of reality. They were devoted to silence and deep contemplation. They wrote ancient texts of truth called *Veda*. These texts may have been produced thousands of years before the Egyptian pyramids were constructed.[7]

Their simple position was that, "Everything comes from the mind. It projects the world exactly as a movie projector does. Our bodies are part of that movie and so is everything that happens to the body."[8]

Now I became very serious about what I put into my mind and about what was said to me about my illness. I tried to stop conversing with people who did

---

[6] Ibid. p. 30.
[7] Ibid. pp. 167-168.
[8] Ibid. p. 183.

not believe that one could heal from EI. I asked my relatives to make a point of mentioning any improvement they noticed. Throughout the day, I repeated, "Every day in every way, I am getting better and better."

I had a lot of work to do and a big illness to heal. It was time for me to learn and use hypnosis regularly.

Chapter 17

HELPING WITH HYPNOSIS

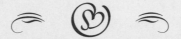

*T*he leaves were turning to golden tones—fall had clearly arrived in New England. My understanding about Environmental Illness was evolving. It was becoming apparent to me that the power to heal was within myself if I could only reach deep inside. Learning the new techniques, such as muscle testing and TAT™, helped me to work at home to encourage the healing process. This suddenly gave me a sense of power and control—*I* could play a key role in this venture! Hypnosis would now be a major contribution to my healing goal.

I had been dabbling in hypnosis since I began studying it in May. I had read many books, written papers, and I was understanding the process. I decided to customize a program. Hypnosis is a serious treatment—the subconscious is powerful and can make many alterations in the body. It was necessary to work correctly and consistently with this new tool.

In this chapter, I will explain how I developed a program of hypnosis. I would like you to understand the reasons and the logic for the selections. Following this explanation, I will outline a suggested hypnosis program that can assist the beginner to become empowered and construct a home therapy session of self-hypnosis. This can be your first step in taking serious control and giving clear positive direction to your wonderful subconscious that you wish to heal and be happy on this great and beautiful earth once again. This is one way you may begin to *reclaim your life!*

If you decide that hypnosis is interesting to you, you may wish to seek the assistance of a professional hypnotherapist. This could be very beneficial. However, I caution, *the therapist should read this book first to understand the level he/she must work at. The standard suggestions can be too strong for a very sensitive individual.* It is a very gentle process that is required to usher the person toward radiant glowing health.

A thorough hypnosis session is comprised of several sections. The logic of each part will now be explained. The seven sections are:

1. Progressive Relaxation
2. Deepening the Relaxation
3. A Special Healing Section
4. End-Result Imagery
5. Posthypnotic Suggestion
6. General Suggestions
7. Counting-Out

Designing the Session

My hypnosis plan first required a relaxation technique—an easy and gentle technique called a passive progressive relaxation. This entailed beginning at the head and suggesting that the muscles in that area relax completely. The technique involves working down the body and suggesting that each area relax totally. The movement progresses from the head and gradually arrives at the toes. This first section begins the relaxation of the body in preparation for further suggestions.

I practiced this a few times to get the feeling of it. It seemed to be simple and very relaxing. I referred to a model from Dr. Krasner's book, *The Wizard Within*. This book was a very helpful guide and I found that I often selected Dr. Krasner's methods for many of my hypnosis sessions.

The next step to consider was a deepening procedure. For this, I decided on a very commonly used technique of going down five steps on a flight of stairs. As I went down the steps, I suggested that I become "deeper and deeper relaxed." As I reached step number one, I became deeply and totally relaxed.

After I perfected this section of the session, I was ready to develop the healing work. At this point, I created a special part entitled, the "Angel of Healing." I suggested that I was lying beside the ocean on a beach I loved. A healing angel with golden hands and fingers came to me. As she touched each area of my body, she brought energy and strength to that area. Then, very gradually I suggested that she touch the areas I wished to heal—basically every part I could think of in my entire body! This part of the healing was my favorite, for it felt so peaceful and wonderful.

The fourth section required a type of imagery— the subconscious responds well to pictures. Visualization sends a clear message to the subconscious mind. I wished for my subconscious to know that I definitely wanted to become well again. I realized that I had been sending very negative messages inward during my illness, because I had been picturing my own funeral. And when I say picturing, I mean picturing! I saw my friends there, my family, the flowers, everything! I had been doing an excellent job of imagining the worst and my subconscious was helping me achieve my goal. Perhaps that was one reason why I kept getting sicker and sicker. I understood now that if I wanted to get well I could not ever do that again.

For my imagery, I selected end-result imagery. The book, *Visualization: The Uses of Imagery in the Health Professions,* written by Errol Korn and Karen Johnson, describes many types of visualizations that can be used. The authors state, "We believe that the most powerful imagery is end-result imagery; that is, developing as clear a picture as is possible of the goal or desired outcome."[1]

During this section, I pictured myself completely well. I began seeing vividly how I was dressed and what I was doing. I imagined myself smiling and I even saw David holding my hand happily and proudly, for I was well. It was a wonderful scene. I even noticed that each time I practiced it, the scene might change. Sometimes I saw myself at the ocean in the sunlight. Other times I visualized myself singing again. Whatever I saw, it felt wonderful and it filled me with hope. Most of all, it sent a clear message to my subconscious about my goal.

Step five involved the insertion of a posthypnotic suggestion to prepare me for the next session. I told myself that the next time I wished to return to this deep state of relaxation, I needed only to rest in a

---

[1] **Chapter 17:** Errol N. Korn and Karen Johnson, *Visualization: The Uses of Imagery in the Health Professions* (Homewood, IL: Dow Jones-Irwin, 1983), 85.

comfortable position, return to the set of five steps, and count down from five to one. When this idea is set, it facilitates the relaxation process.

Section six of the program is the suggestion portion. This allowed me to issue direct ideas about my healing. This is a very helpful and important part. Suggestions can render noticeable results; it is important to know how to do this correctly. Because much care needs to be taken, I will explain some of the requirements concerning utilizing suggestions about healing. The knowledge is helpful, but when you are dealing with Environmental Illness, use even more care and attention. Some of the general comments can be too powerful and promote problems for very sensitive people. *Extreme care must be used when making suggestions to sensitive people. The healing must be gentle and well-integrated with that person's psyche.* A person with EI might be very fearful about returning to the world that inflicted the injury. First, a feeling of being safe and the belief that recovery is possible must be achieved.

The subconscious mind possesses certain characteristics that need to be understood before a person can be successful at using hypnotic suggestions. Some of the traits are explained by Dr. Krasner:

The subconscious mind has neither emotion nor opinion. It responds only from the information stored within its memory, retrieving that information very much as you would pull up a letter from a file cabinet. It accepts uncritically all suggestions and ideas given to it by the conscious mind, and it acts upon them with no judgment whatsoever. It cannot differentiate between what is real and what is imagined. No amount of willpower exerted by the conscious mind can override it for any extended time. . . . That is also why hypnosis works. The relaxed state of hypnosis provides easier access to your subconscious mind.[2]

The subconscious mind is very literal and does not contain the critical awareness of the conscious mind. Therefore, if you were to ask a person in a hypnotic state if he/she can count from one to ten, the answer would be "yes," rather than the expected counting. Only the critical mind "figures out" what you really intended. So, when you develop your suggestions, you must realize that the subconscious mind will accept them readily and uncritically. This is a wonderful feature of hypnosis, but it is also a serious factor to consider. You must be careful what you ask of your subconscious. You need to be realistic. You cannot ask it to cure you in one week if you have been sick for many years.

A very important rule in devising suggestions is to use only positive terms. Using negatives is not effective with the subconscious. Instead of saying, "I won't be *afraid* of *chemicals* anymore," you might say instead, "I feel *safe* and *secure* in a *healthy* and *clean environment.*" This is a positive suggestion. If you use the first suggestion, the subconscious will focus on the words *afraid* and *chemicals,* words that will not have a healing effect and may even create the opposite effect of instilling more fear. It is better for the subconscious to hear the words *safe, secure,* and *clean environment.*

Another essential factor is to speak in the present tense. The subconscious mind does not understand

---

[2] A. M. Krasner, Ph.D. *The Wizard Within* (Santa Anna, CA: American Board of Hypnotherapy Press, 1991), 79.

general future suggestions like, "I *will* get better someday." This is too general and too vague. It would be better to say, "Each day I feel healthier and healthier."

It is acceptable to mention specific times in the future—if they are phrased carefully. For example, if you wish to encourage sleep at night, instead of saying, "I will not *stay awake* at *night*," you might say, "At night, I *sleep peacefully* and *calmly, benefiting* from a *deep restful night's sleep.*" In the first statement, the subconscious heard only *stay awake.* In the second suggestion, the subconscious heard *night, sleep, peacefully, calmly,* and so on. The *descriptive* words are very helpful to the subconscious, so be attentive to the image you are creating.

It is also a good idea to repeat the suggestion, because the subconscious responds better if there is some repetition. The idea can be repeated in different words and still convey the same message.[3]

My final caution is that you should go very slowly. First, use only suggestions to feel safe in the world and to say that you are better and better every day. Give the clear intention that your body wishes to heal completely. Also, deal with self-esteem. Something like, "I am a wonderful person healing a wonderful body" can be helpful. Often a person with EI feels unhappy and discouraged about his/her own body, because it has failed. Low self-esteem is often a serious issue.

Building a positive self-image assists the subconscious in focusing on healing and believing that you can heal, and further, that you are worthy of healing.

---

[3] Ibid. pp. 83-90.

Many people with EI think that they need to *detoxify, detoxify, detoxify!* Be very cautious about suggesting this to your subconscious. Once, I purchased a general healing hypnosis tape. The therapist on it suggested, "Release anything blocking you from perfect health." The next day I felt very sick. My body reacted poorly to that suggestion. The subconscious could not perform that task—it was not realistic. Someone with EI has much to release. It may be emotions, traumas, and physical toxins. To simply suggest that all blocks be released can be unhealthy. The subconscious knows no boundaries. It will attempt to accomplish it all at once. It may be too much! In my case, my subconscious balked at it and reacted badly.

At first, it is not even a good idea to suggest releasing anything. Allow your body to accept that it can heal and become totally well. This process may take a few weeks or a few months. When it does adjust to that concept, then, very gradually and gently, you can suggest that you release any emotions that are safe for you to release and that you are ready to release. You should also include that you feel comfortable and that the emotions are released at a safe pace and through the proper emotional channels.

If you wish to release toxins, you would issue the same suggestion in the same manner—"at a safe pace so that it is comfortable for my body, and by way of the proper elimination channels." Always be careful about forming your suggestions. Listen to what you are asking your subconscious to do. Hear your words literally as if a child were listening. If you clarify your request so that it is exactly what you want to happen, it will be to your benefit.

Because you are new at forming suggestions, an initial sentence at the beginning of the suggestion portion can protect your subconscious from any destructive idea you might accidentally put forth. A statement like, "I only accept those suggestions that are for my ultimate good, and my healing goal" serves that purpose nicely.

Once you understand the principles of self-hypnosis, you can prepare a tape for yourself. A tape is a good idea because you can write your script in advance, making sure you are suggesting appropriate pictures and ideas. Then you record it. After that, you may sit back and totally relax. You know there will be no unexpected surprises and you can feel safe in the comfort of your own home.

However, you need to remember to revise the suggestions from time to time as you heal, so that the suggestions match your changing symptoms and needs. This may involve a lot of work and be very time-consuming, but the results make it worth the effort.

If you choose to make your own tape, speak in a soft, lilting voice, pausing between thoughts. Be totally relaxed as you speak to convey a relaxed energy.

If it is your own voice on the tape, then you should use the pronoun "I." For example, say, "As I become stronger each day, I feel safer and safer on this earth." This will create a deep connection between yourself and your psyche. You can become your own "best friend."

Hypnosis Suggestions for Environmental Illness

Listed below are some possible suggestions you might use when dealing with Environmental Illness. The following suggestions are only possibilities, but you might understand the concept better if you see actual suggestions. Select five suggestions; it is best to focus on only one or two goals. If you work on too many ideas, your attention is divided and the effect may be weakened.

The following sentences are phrased using the pronoun "I," which is what you will use when recording your tape.

- *I only accept those suggestions that are for my ultimate good and my healing goal.*

- *I take excellent care of my health. I eat nutritious food for my body, and I use hypnosis to direct my mind toward my healing goal. I love healing my body and mind.*

- *As I think more positive thoughts, my body becomes healthier and healthier. My body loves it when I am optimistic and happy.*

- *I am more and more positive about my future. I see myself well and happy. Every cell and fiber of my being rejoices at the wonderful prospect of perfect, glowing health, and a happy life filled with ease and peace.*

- *As I become stronger, I feel safer and safer on this earth. I become calm and secure, knowing that I am healing and gaining strength.*

- *I want to be totally present on this earth. I am happy to be included in life's experiences. It feels wonderful to be totally present on this earth.*

- *At night, I sleep peacefully through the night. I benefit from a restful, calm night's sleep. It feels wonderful to sleep deeply and comfortably through the night.*

- *I relax on all levels knowing that I am healing. It is an excellent feeling to move closer and closer to perfect glowing health.*

- *I am a wonderful person healing a wonderful body. I deserve perfect vibrant health.*

- *I allow myself to release my illness at a comfortable pace that is safe for my body. It is time to move toward a life of health and happiness.*

- *Step by step, I walk away from my past condition and move closer and closer to excellent glowing health. This feels wonderful for my body, and I am happy to be healthy and strong.*

- *Every day in every way, I am getting better and better, healthier and healthier, and stronger and stronger.*

Please notice some repetition contained in the sentences. This helps to reach the subconscious. If the issue is very important, more repetition might be necessary. Most of all, see how each statement is optimistic and has positive adjectives. There are no negative words—these should be strictly avoided in this circumstance.

Please note that the issue of detoxification has not yet been addressed. Later, after the subconscious has accepted the idea that you can get well and you will be safe doing so, then you can encourage the body to release toxins and emotions. Here are some healing suggestions:

- *I allow myself to release any toxins I am ready to release through the proper elimination channels, at a comfortable rate, and at a rate that is safe for my body. My organs remain balanced while my healing process occurs.*

- *I allow myself to release any emotions I need to release through the proper elimination channels, at a comfortable rate, and at a rate that is*

*safe for my body. My organs remain balanced
while this healing process occurs.*

These are important suggestions and need to be carefully given. It is important to work cautiously with a
sensitive person, always mentioning that the healing
process occurs at a safe rate. The individual must be
able to adjust to the changes that result. If he feels
too uncomfortable, he might become frightened;
blocks to the healing process may occur.

A session of this length may be enjoyed once a
week. It is not necessary to repeat the work too often—the subconscious has heard you and will then
process the requests. Allow for this inner work. A
very sensitive person needs to permit the adjustment
and deal with the changes hypnosis creates. Once a
week is fine if it is a well-structured session. The subconscious will love the assistance and thrive on the
positive suggestions.

You may even observe that your self-talk during
the week begins to change and becomes more positive. This happens gradually, but it is a nice benefit
of hypnosis. Eventually, when you hear others speaking negatively about healing, you will notice it immediately. It will seem very foreign to you.

Counting-Out

A last and very important part of the hypnosis session is the counting-out portion. If you have achieved
a nice relaxed state, you will need to make sure that
you come out properly. You may suggest that you are
going to count from one to five. When you reach number five, you will be wide awake, clear-headed, and
relaxed. Exact words you may utilize are included in
the outline at the end of this chapter.

When this portion is done properly, you should feel well after the session. It is advisable to count out slowly, allowing your body to make the shift back into the normal waking state with ease and comfort. The body needs to adjust. So, as in everything I speak about, the key word is *gently.* Do these changes *GENTLY.*

Hypnosis is a wonderful tool to access a deep level of healing. If used wisely and carefully, it can render marvelous results.

Outline-Sample Hypnosis Session

I. **Passive Progressive Relaxation**—At the opening of the session, state your intention for that particular healing time. Be clear and concise. This assists your wonderful subconscious to understand your plan. Follow this by gradually and gently directing your body to relax progressively from your head to your feet.

It is my intention to reach a deep level of relaxation and to access my inner ability of healing. I wish to feel deep inner peace and to allow my body to understand that I can heal and become totally present on this earth. (Vary this depending on your personal intention for this session.)

Now I bring my attention to my head. I relax the muscles in my head—allowing all tension to leave my head. I completely relax my head.

I move to my eyes—closing them gently. Letting go of tension and relaxing my eyes.

I move to my cheeks and relax my cheeks and my face muscles. I release any tension and relax my face muscles.

I focus on my jaw. I allow my mouth to open ever so slightly . . . allowing all tension and stress to leave my jaw and relaxing that area totally.

I breathe deeply and relax. (Take a soothing deep breath here.) *With each deep breath I take during this session, I relax more and more.*

Now I bring my attention to my neck. I relax all the muscles in my neck . . . letting go of all tension and stress held in my neck . . . relaxing the muscles and relaxing my neck.

I move to my shoulders and totally relax my shoulders. I let them drop and let all tension and stress go away as I completely relax my shoulders. It feels wonderful to totally relax my shoulders.

I focus on my chest. I let all tension float up out of my chest . . . I relax the muscles in my chest. Breathing and relaxing.

I direct my attention to my abdominal area. I release the tension in the abdominal muscles and relax. I allow all tension and stress to leave that area . . . relaxing.

I move to my back and I relax my back muscles. I allow the tension to leave my back, so that it is completely and totally relaxed. My lower back feels relaxed and peaceful.

Breathing deeply and relaxing.

I focus on my arms and allow all tension to leave my upper arms . . . relaxing the muscles in my upper arms. Then focus on my lower arms . . . allowing all the tension to move down my arms, as it moves out of my body. I let it move into my hands and out my fingers . . . all the tension and stress gone from that area . . . out my fingers and away.

Breathing deeply and relaxing.

Now I bring my attention to my upper legs. I allow all tension and stress to leave that area . . . moving down the legs to the lower legs . . . down to the feet . . . and gradually out through the toes. All tension and stress out the toes and away . . . leaving my legs and feet completely and totally relaxed.

Now I scan my body and notice any area that might still be tense . . . perhaps my neck . . . perhaps my shoulders or my abdomen—any area where I may feel tension or strain. I release the tension in this area so that my body can be completely and totally relaxed.

Breathing and relaxing. It feels wonderful to be deeply relaxed of all levels. It is a perfectly natural and healthy state.

At this point you should be feeling calmer. You are now prepared for the deepening suggestions that will lead you to a very relaxed state.

II. **Deepening Procedure**—This section can be easily presented by using five steps. Proceed slowly. The following words can give you an idea of simple deepening suggestions.

I am picturing five steps. I am standing on step number five. As I count down the steps, I become deeper and deeper relaxed. When I reach step

*number one, I will be completely and deeply
relaxed. I begin on step number **Five** . . . Now
I step down . . . slowly down . . . to step number
Four . . . becoming more relaxed . . . Now I step
down to step number **Three** . . . into deeper relaxation . . . Slowly down. I step down to step
number **Two**. As I stand on step number **Two**, I
am becoming more and more relaxed . . . And
now step down to step number **One** . . . deeply,
deeply relaxed . . . completely and totally relaxed.*

III. **Special Healing Section**—This is a portion I
devised to encourage inner healing. If it res-
onates with you, you may wish to give it a try.

*I place myself in a beautiful setting where I feel
completely safe and secure. The air is crystal
clear and I feel wonderful. There are delicate
white fluffy clouds drifting softly by. A bird in
the distance is singing a song of good luck and
good fortune. I hear the ocean surf beside me.
I am given a soft silky bed to lie upon, and a
golden robe to adorn my body for this healing
experience. The Angel of Healing comes to my
side. She has beautiful golden hands and fingers. Gently and lovingly, she touches various
parts of my body. As she touches each location,
she opens the energy meridians so that the area
may receive sufficient energy to work perfectly.
She brings energy and strength to each area
she touches.*

Select the locations of your body you wish to
strengthen. It is a good idea to include the organs and glands, tissues and cells. Here is how
you may wish to direct this process.

She gently touches my head. She clears away the worries and fears, which have troubled me for so long. My brain receives oxygen and a healthy blood supply, so that I think clearly and my memory improves.

She moves to my eyes, so that I see clearly. My eyes are strong and healthy. Light enters easily and feels wonderful.

She touches my ears. They hear beautifully. Sound enters easily and feels wonderful.

Then she touches my sinus area. She heals the mucous membranes within, so that I breathe clear fresh air and filter out allergens efficiently. My sinuses are calm and comfortable.

She moves to my neck and shoulders. She brings ease and relaxation to this area. I feel completely relaxed in my neck and shoulders.

She touches my chest area. The tissues are clear and healthy there.

Gently and lovingly, she moves to my heart and it is beating regularly and perfectly, for my maximum health. The arteries are clear and healthy.

The Angel of Healing touches my lungs and they breathe beautifully, bringing fresh air and oxygen to my body. They breathe clearly and openly.

She moves to my liver and touches it ever so gently. She gives it extra special loving care, so that the energy opens to that area and the liver works efficiently, filtering out toxins and performing all its functions perfectly.

She touches my spleen, so that it filters my blood as it should.

She moves to my pancreas and touches it gently, so that it functions perfectly for me.

She touches my gall bladder, bringing it strength and health.

She moves to my stomach, helping it digest beautifully.

She moves to my small intestine and large intestine, so that they are strong and healthy for me. She strengthens the probiotic intestinal flora within.

Very gently, she touches my kidneys, bladder, and urinary tract, bringing energy to the entire area, so each part works perfectly and easily for the health of my body.

She touches my glands, so that they work in a balanced fashion, harmoniously, for the good of the entire body.

And ever so gently with her golden hands of healing, she moves over the tissues and cells, helping them to heal and renew.

My organs remain balanced while the healing process occurs.

She smiles, for all parts are working in perfect harmony throughout my body . . . healing and working together for the ultimate good of my body.

Wonderful!

This is a sample. Please notice that I have not been very specific about the correct functioning of each part; the subconscious knows perfectly well how each area operates. It is only necessary to suggest that the part return to perfect harmony within the body.

Other special healing images can also be utilized. An idea of liquid light gently moving down the body may be enjoyable. Each area it touches becomes soothed and strengthened. This is acceptable if a person tolerates light well. If you happen to be light sensitive, avoid this type of imagery.

Along with the benefits of strengthening your body, this section will relax you further—deepening the hypnotic state.

IV. **End-Result Imagery**—This section is very important: you guide your subconscious with imagery. The subconscious responds well to pictures, so now is the time to utilize this powerful tool to direct your healing.

I see myself completely well. I am doing an activity I enjoy. My clothes are lovely. I see the outfit I am wearing and even the exact color. I notice the shoes on my feet. I am smiling and the expression on my face is one of strength and confidence—I am healthy and I welcome this joyous result. I see my friends and they, too, are smiling, for they are proud of me for my healing journey. I see the setting around me. I am well and it feels wonderful! I can go anywhere I want and do anything I wish to do, for I am well and strong. I am totally present on the earth and it feels wonderful. My energy meridians remain open when other energy fields merge with mine. It feels excellent to be open and clear.

At the count of three I take a photograph of this scene. 1 . . . 2 . . . 3 . . . click. Now I see myself placing this picture in a photo album for my wonderful subconscious. The album is entitled (your name)—Completely Well. I invite my subconscious to refer to this photograph collection to see that this is how I wish to be—healthy and happy on this earth. I ask to be guided in this direction gradually and at a rate that is safe for my body.

Each time you experience this visualization, you might find that you picture a different scene. This is perfectly fine, for a variety of wonderful images will render marvelous results within the subconscious and they will be amusing to place in your special photograph album!

V. **Posthypnotic Suggestion**—The addition of a posthypnotic suggestion will facilitate your relaxation for the next session.

The next time I wish to return to this deep and wonderful state of relaxation, I only need to rest in a comfortable position and picture the set of five steps. As I count from five down to one— when I reach step number one, I will be deeply and totally relaxed.

VI. **Suggestions for Healing**—Now you must be very careful to suggest only those ideas that are realistic and clear. To protect against any mistake you may make, begin with this statement, "I only accept those suggestions that are for my ultimate good and my healing goal." Then proceed with suggestions concerning positive changes you need at the time. Some samples are already within the chapter. A few additional ones might be:

Each day I eat nutritious food and take very good care of my body. I love healing my wonderful body.

My NAET™ treatments clear easily and completely. It is wonderful to clear my allergies and sensitivities.

And don't forget my favorite statement, a variation of Emile Coué's positive words!

Every day in every way I am getting stronger and stronger, healthier and healthier.

Focus on just what you wish to accomplish at the time and CAREFULLY compose your suggestions.

VII. Counting-Out—This is a very important section. Proceed slowly and gently to bring yourself back to the normal waking state.

I will count from one to five. When I reach number five, I will be wide awake, clear-headed, and relaxed. Slowly begin counting to five. **One**— *ever so gently beginning to wake up.* **Two**— *waking up more and more.* **Three**—*moving my fingers and toes.* **Four**—*body processes returning to normal.* **Five**—*wide awake, wide awake, clear-headed, relaxed, and wide awake!*

You may find that you need to rest after your session, for your body has been deeply relaxed. Enjoy the inner peace you feel. You have just gently ushered your body another step closer toward perfect, glowing health.

Although I constantly worked with hypnosis to be positive and determined, there were often roadblocks placed before me. It was as if there were a path of healing with brambles and thorns every so often just to test my fortitude! Once again I was about to encounter a major hurdle and would have to muster the strength to continue on and travel forward toward my healing goal.

Chapter 18

BAD NEWS

*T*his fall marked two years since my injury in 1994. September had become a very stressful time of year for me. It was a sore reminder that I could not return to school like everybody else. I felt terrible. However, I tried to focus on the fact that I had at least found a doctor who was finally helping me. It had taken me nearly two years to find him, but thank goodness I had.

By early October, I had not yet heard the judge's decision on my worker's compensation. Still only receiving 45 percent of my pay, we were barely able to pay the bills. I kept hoping I would hear soon that he had decided to award me 60 percent, which is full compensation. It was still much less than I would have been making if I had been able to work, but it would have helped. Then, one day the envelope arrived. My hands trembled as I opened it. I had to open it cautiously because particles in the air could give me a breathing problem. I held my breath so as not to inhale any fibers of paper.

After placing it under the glass reading table, I began to read. The initial words brought encouragement.

The judge was saying that my husband and I were very credible witnesses. He did believe that I was totally disabled. He also believed that the disability had begun at the time of the exposure. But then the message began to change. He continued on. Since the disability had not gone away on December 31, 1994 and was still going on, it must not be related to the roofing fumes. I had to read this statement over again. I couldn't believe what I was reading! The judge had taken the side of Dr. Kane, the "impartial" doctor, paid for by the Board of Industrial Accidents. It was he who had decided that I should have completely recovered from the exposure to the fumes by December 31. He even predicted the exact day that I should have awakened well! The judge actually listened to him and disregarded my own doctors' opinions, whom I had been seeing for over a year and a half. Instead he took the side of this "impartial" man whom I had seen for one hour and who didn't believe in MCS!

I began to tremble. What would this mean? I was almost afraid to continue reading. Then I read on. The judge had decided that I deserved no compensation. I was shocked. Then I continued. The next part I truly couldn't believe. Not only did he decide that I deserved no compensation, but now he was ordering me to pay back all the compensation he had awarded me in the first place! Anything paid to me after December 31, the magical date Dr. Kane had decreed as the day of recovery, was to be returned.

My entire body began to shake. I was so frightened. How could this be? I had been so injured by the fumes. They had rendered me unable to work anywhere or even take care of myself. I was so vulnerable and now I was being deserted! Without any salary at all and thousands of dollars in medical bills, I was supposed to pay back the money the judge had awarded me—money already used to pay some of the extensive bills. I felt sick.

I started pacing the floor. I was wringing my hands and my body was weak. I didn't know what to do. Why had the insurance company spent so much money trying to deny my compensation? They had attempted to conduct surveillance to see if I was going places and if this was a fraudulent claim. The man sent to do this task had been unable to complete it; he reported that, "Mrs. Smith never left her home." Doesn't this tell them something about my condition? Then they paid for lawyers and the laughing doctor twice! All that money spent to keep me from receiving what my employer paid into the fund for injured employees. What was this all about? That money they spent to take away my rights could have helped me in so many ways. It could have paid some of my vast medical bills!

When David arrived home, I was still pacing. I was dizzy and feeling sick. He asked me what was wrong. I handed him the papers. He began to read. He went quietly into the den. When he came back into the kitchen, he was pale. He was also upset and he was angry. He couldn't understand why they would refuse me when I was so very sick and obviously injured by the fumes. He went into the other room and sat alone. I don't know what was going on inside his head; he stayed there for a long time. When he returned to the kitchen, he sat by me. Gently, he comforted me, "Please, don't worry. Everything is going to be all right." I knew he was scared about our future. He had always tried to reassure me, but that night I thought he was trying to calm himself.

Then I began to cry. I told him I was so sorry for getting hurt. I had ruined everything. Now we could lose our home that we had been paying the mortgage on for many years. I was so distressed. I wanted to help him in some way, but I was just not able to earn any money. The tears flowed and flowed. He held me and rocked me. I think he wanted to cry too, but he held it in. He was so brave.

I slept very little that night. I woke up exhausted. My appointment with Doctor Sampson was that morning and I didn't want to miss it. Every treatment was so desperately needed. David drove me and we talked about what we were going to do. He didn't know how he would pay back the debt the judge had imposed. I felt sick. It required great effort to remain calm for David and to prepare for my treatment.

When we arrived at Robert and Patricia's, we were glum. With slumped shoulders and swollen eyes, I walked into the treatment room. The moment I looked into Robert's kind eyes, I broke down into tears again. He tried to comfort me. Patricia came in. They were so kind and understanding. I just kept remarking that I could not believe how shabbily I was being treated. Why was I being deserted like this? I felt as if I were being left by the side of the road to die. Nobody cared! The only efforts being put forth were those meant to avoid any responsibility. For twenty years I had given so much of my energy to being the best teacher I could be. I had never asked for anything in my life before. The one time I needed help, everyone—the school, the doctor, the insurance company, and the court—just coldly turned their backs!

Robert was very concerned. He didn't think I should receive a treatment that day. This disappointed me. I promised that I would calm down. After steadying myself, and regaining my composure, a treatment was administered.

When we returned home, there was a message from my attorney. He expressed his shock at the unfair decision. He reiterated that this had been such a strong case. Perhaps that was the problem. He had been so very confident that the facts would carry themselves. He allowed me to see Dr. Kane, who, he knew ahead of time, didn't believe in MCS. Also, my lawyer had confided that he hadn't even prepared for my first hearing until the day before it was scheduled. I suddenly understood that the case couldn't take care of itself. I had just been too sick to realize that my lawyer was also avoiding his responsibility.

Now it was too late to rectify the mistake. The decision was rendered. I had to find another lawyer and try to get some help to secure my Accidental Disability Retirement. If I lost that as well, I would have nothing for the rest of my life!

So, the quest for a new attorney began and I tried to focus on my healing once again. I just couldn't think too much about this defeat, for I couldn't risk going back downhill.

In order to receive my Accidental Disability Retirement, I was required to be examined by three doctors selected by the Teachers' Retirement Board. A vote of two out of the three was necessary to allow the board to grant a pension. That same month, I was assigned to see two of the doctors. I felt discouraged. Would this be another fiasco? Would these doctors also laugh at me and say that there is no such illness? I wasn't sure that I could take any more mockery.

Reluctantly, I went to the first doctor. He was a well-known specialist in the area of MCS. When he met me, he showed genuine concern. He told me I was suffering too much. He even suggested that after my retirement was decided, I should see him as my doctor so that he might help me with some of my problems. I was relieved. This man knew about MCS. He understood how terrible my life was. I left feeling that at least there were doctors who cared. If only there were more of them.

Three weeks later, I went to the second doctor I had been assigned to. He, too, was a specialist in Boston. He also was dismayed when he saw me. He shook his head and said that I was the fourth person that month whom he had seen with MCS, inflicted from roofing fumes!

Both these doctors wrote very long, comprehensive reports detailing the injury and the resultant illness. They believed very strongly that I had been and continued to be injured by the fumes. MCS is a real and very disabling condition. At last! A vote of two out of three doctors was all that was necessary to receive my pension. I was getting a little hopeful. Now I only needed a good attorney to represent me and maybe, just maybe . . .

Joan, the leader of the support group, informed me about a woman attorney who was familiar with MCS. When we conversed on the phone, I was impressed with her knowledge of the illness and her intelligence. She agreed to come to my house; she realized that it would be very difficult for me to travel to her office in Boston. I was a little reluctant, because I had not had anybody in my home except for my mother and my husband since the injury. She insisted that she knew how to prepare for me. She promised not to wear any fragrance or dry-cleaned clothes. Hesitantly, I agreed. I knew that even a shampoo or deodorant with fragrance could still be difficult for me. But, I needed a new lawyer. I opened all the windows and hoped for the best.

When she arrived, I did fairly well. She took off her coat and handed it to me. Little did she realize that I was sensitive to fabrics and I immediately began to react. I took the wool coat and quickly placed it on my couch in the living room. I left the room and accompanied her to the kitchen. I managed to be with her in my house. I sat away from her and we

talked about my case. She informed me that I could
not appeal the worker's compensation decision, because if I lost, I would not be able to continue to pur-
sue my Accidental Disability Retirement. There were
so many rules! So, I had to settle the case. I agreed,
because my pension was very important to me. I had
paid into this retirement plan for twenty years.

After our meeting, she agreed to take on my case.
I would pay her by the hour. She charged a large sum,
but David and I figured that if she devoted enough
time to my case, perhaps we might win.

There was much to do, but I was, at least, doing
my best. One additional doctor remained to be seen
before I could have a hearing with the board. It took
several months before this was scheduled. When I
went to this man, I discovered that he was a trained
anesthesiologist! He had done some course work in
the area of environmental issues, but his specialty
was clearly anesthesiology. He arrived for the appointment wearing after-shave lotion! This posed
great difficulty, so I asked him if he had a room with
a window. He said that he did and ushered me to another room. It had a plate glass window that didn't
open. When I inquired about that, he replied that he
hadn't realized that I needed to open it! Did he think
I needed a *nice view?* What was this man thinking?

Then while I was discussing the effects of my injury, I mentioned that I had not seen a friend in
years. He asked me what was wrong with *my
friends!* I knew I was going to have a problem with
this man. He had no clue about the illness. So, when
his report arrived, it reflected this. Still, he admitted
that I was totally disabled. He just didn't know why.
So, at least I had the other two doctors for my necessary vote. I would wait for the hearing. Perhaps
this time I had a chance.

PART III

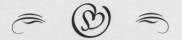

The course has been set. I must not falter or allow distractions to bar my way. I listen closely as God whispers to me. It is a long way over the obstacles and much work needs to be done.

Chapter 19

ARE YOU WILLING?

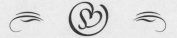

*I*n spite of this tiring month dealing with my financial concerns, I continued to make small improvements. They were subtle, but they were real. My body felt stronger all over. I even found an old pair of cotton slacks and a sweater I could wear. Now I had another outfit to alternate with my old worn-out gray clothes. This would be the third winter in that *lovely* ensemble and I wasn't sure it would last. I appreciated it for keeping me warm, but I so wanted to wear my other clothes again!

I also could use my den. Now I was able to be in two rooms downstairs. I could even sit in my easy chair and recline. It felt so luxurious to sit in a comfortable chair. For two years, I had only been able to sit in a hard chair all day. I could never rest during the day.

I went regularly to Dr. Sampson and Patricia every week. I learned more and more from Robert. He seemed to know so much about energetic healing. One week he introduced me to a new concept. It was called being "100 percent willing." This turned out to be one of my favorite techniques and extremely helpful to me in my healing.

It was very difficult for me to conceive that a person who is seriously ill can actually have blocks, at some level, to his or her own healing process. How could I want to remain allergic? Yet, when Robert tested me, I would test weak when I made certain statements, meaning that I indeed had a block about healing.

At first Robert used this technique on me, but soon I started experimenting with it at home. I found that, concerning most things I had difficulty with, there was usually a block at some level. My body had some resistance to letting the problem go. Now I understand this more—once a person has Environmental Illness, it becomes an overwhelming task to be willing to heal and go back out into the world that has destroyed so much. I knew that I was angry, sad, and frightened. I had lost so much and was suffering. I began to realize that these emotions needed to be released somehow. Just speaking about them wasn't enough. Also, I probably wasn't even aware of some of them held deep within.

So, this technique, devised by Dr. Bruce Dewe and his wife Joan Dewe was written about in their book, *Professional Kinesiology Practice II: Advanced Specialized Kinesiology Methods.* As usual, Dr. Sampson knew very well how to use it and he taught it to me.

I will explain how I used it at home. By using this technique, you can clear out the blocks and allow any treatment to be more effective. Even the NAET™ treatments sometimes didn't clear for me until I did my "100 percent willing" treatment.

First, you phrase a statement with these initial words, "I am 100 percent willing to give up the need . . ." To finish the statement you decide what item you wish to work on. Let's use, for example, a certain allergy. How about milk? We would complete the statement with . . . " to have an allergy to milk." Now we have a statement, "I'm 100 percent willing to give up the need to have an allergy to milk."

Next, you muscle test after you say this statement. If you test weak, you have a block at some level about giving up your allergy to milk.

The **next step** is to see what level is involved. You ask, "Is it physical, emotional, social, mental, spiritual, financial, or any other level known or unknown?" You muscle test as you say each level. Usually, one of these will go weak and you will have established the level. Let's say it's the physical level for example. Keep that in mind—*physical*. We'll come back to that later.

Then go on to find out what element is involved. These elements come from the Oriental model of health. They are Earth, Water, Fire, Wood, and Metal. Also Dr. and Mrs. Dewe have added Central Vessel and Governing Vessel. As you ask about each element, you muscle test. When one of the elements tests weak, you have established the element involved. For our example, let's say the element *wood* goes weak.

The **final step** is to determine the emotion. The Dewes list some emotions for each element. Once you know what element is involved, you only need to question the emotions under that element. Basically the emotions for the elements are as follows:

> **Earth:** empathy, sympathy
>
> **Water:** anxiety, fear, terror
>
> **Fire:** love, joy, hate
>
> **Wood:** anger, rage, wrath

Metal: guilt, grief, regret

Central Vessel: success, respect, overwhelmed

Governing Vessel: trust, support, honesty

Now, since the element was *wood,* we ask, "Is it anger, rage, wrath?" We push as we say each emotion. When one goes weak, we have the emotion involved. Now let's say that *wrath* went weak.

Earlier, we established that our problem is at the *physical* level. Now we know that the element is *wood* and the emotion is *wrath.* This is all you need to use to clear the block. Actually, you don't need to mention the element any longer. You only need to focus on the *physical* level and *wrath.*

It is not necessary to analyze *why* you feel *wrath* over this issue or why it is the *physical* level. This clearing takes place on an energetic level and happens quickly and easily, without the need to dwell on the reasons. Simply take the pose I will now explain and the block can be cleared.

Sit quietly and place your right hand across your forehead. Place your left hand behind your head at its base. Your hands should be in a horizontal position with the floor. Be sure your legs are not crossed. (See Fig. 3.)

Then **think quietly,** "Lack of 100 percent willingness to give up my need to be allergic to milk, physical level, wrath."

Say this to yourself three times. That is usually enough. You can experiment. Then you stand up, bring your hands down to your sides, and say the original statement to see if it has cleared: "I'm 100 percent willing to give up my need to have an allergy to milk."

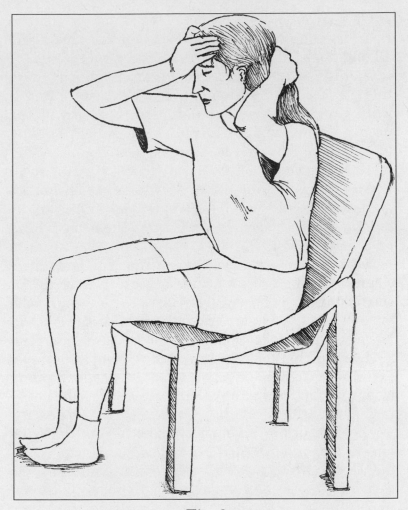

Fig. 3

When you test, the muscle should be strong. This means you have cleared the block to the allergy. After this clearing, it is easier to eliminate the allergy with the NAET™. Sometimes, my allergy went away with just this clearing.

Often, when dealing with a troublesome allergy or serious issue, it is possible to get an answer such

as, "all levels, all emotions." This is no problem to
clear. Assume the pose and focus on "all levels and
all emotions."

Additionally, after the first statement is cleared,
there is a second statement. It is "I'm 100 percent
willing to *accept the positive benefits* of giving up the
need . . ." This is slightly different from the first. You
follow the procedure the same way as the first statement, using the exact final part to the statement. In
this case, it is, "to have an allergy to milk." The entire
statement would be, "I'm 100 percent willing to *accept the positive benefits* of giving up the need to have
an allergy to milk."

Usually, however, you may find that you have
cleared for the second statement after clearing for
the first. Only rarely will you have to go through the
entire procedure again. But if it is necessary, it will
be very beneficial to completely clear the block.

I found this tool (100 percent willing technique)
extremely supportive and it gradually helped me to
clear any blocks and any emotions that might be interfering with my healing. It is indicated if a specific
allergy is stuck or an emotion is bothering you. This
effective technique clears the block on the appropriate level. Often, you will notice the results of the
clearing. If it is an emotion, you will not be bothered
by it after the clearing. If it is an allergy, you may
see it clear easily with a NAET™ treatment or all by
itself.

You might wonder what areas of concern can be
covered with this technique. Basically anything you
are having trouble with in your life can be dealt
with using this technique. Some possible statements might be, "I'm 100 percent willing to give up
the need . . .

to have asthma."
to have allergies."
to have sensitivities to chemicals."
to be unable to eat fruit."
to have a problem with my thyroid."
to be angry with my friend."
to worry about my friend."
to lose sleep at night."

As you can see, many types of problems can be addressed with this procedure. They can be health issues, allergies, emotional problems, or any other life situations where you feel you are blocked.

If perhaps you might be resisting and thinking, "Oh no, not me, I wouldn't block my own energy," just try a few and see how weak you may test for the statement and then how strong you test afterward. It is a surprise for most people. I know it took me a while to accept this realization.

You may also be wondering how many issues may be cleared at one time. Usually, one or two clearings of both statements are recommended. Do not exceed this amount unless you are being treated by a trained kinesiologist. Also, it is advisable to ask your body if it is appropriate to work on another item "at this time." Remember, each clearing requires processing time. It is important to proceed carefully.

If you just follow the steps and work with them, the procedure becomes easier after awhile. It provided me with another tool to control my illness and a way to help myself during the week when the problems would occur. Also, my handy tool of muscle testing guided me in finding the answers.

Here is a brief summary of this technique.

One Hundred Percent Willing

I. **Say the statement,** "I'm 100 percent willing to give up the need to . . ." Finish the statement with the problem or allergy that is stuck.

II. **Muscle test** (refer to Chapter 13) to see if the arm goes weak. If this occurs, you need to work on this problem.

III. **Check** to see what level it is (physical, emotional, social, mental, spiritual, financial, or any other level known or unknown).

IV. **Check** to see what element is involved (Earth, Water, Fire, Wood, Metal, Central Vessel, or Governing Vessel).

V. **Check** to see what emotion is involved (see chart in this chapter).

VI. **Sit** in the position described in this chapter, (see Fig. 3) with your right hand across your forehead and your left hand across the back of your head at its base. Do not cross your legs or feet. Say the statement, "Lack of 100 percent willingness to give up the need to . . . (state the problem), (level), and (emotion)." Repeat this three times.

VII. **Stand up** and say the original statement again and muscle test to see if the arm remains strong. If it does, you have cleared the block. If not, you may have to do the entire process over to see if you got the right information.

VIII. **Now check the statement,** "I'm 100 percent willing to accept the positive benefits of giving up the need to . . . " This will probably be clear if you have successfully cleared the original statement. If not, work on it in the exact same fashion as the original statement.[1]

At first, this procedure may seem complicated, but after you become accustomed to the process, it is a very helpful and handy way of assisting yourself to clear blocks and to become healthier. It can make a significant difference on levels you may not have been able to penetrate before. Your body will begin to accept the healing process with more ease and you will begin to feel less resistance within. This is a wonderful technique that has been extremely valuable in my healing process.

Many of these new energy treatments were changing the course of my condition. These wonderful contributions were the result of my association with two special people: Dr. Robert Sampson and Patricia Hughes. I would like to devote a special chapter to them at this time.

---

[1] **Chapter 19:** Bruce A. Dewe, M.D. and Joan R. Dewe, MA. *Professional Kinesiology Pratice II: Advanced Specialised Kinesiology Methods* (Aukland, New Zealand: Professional Health Publications, 1997), 1. PKP 3-year Certification Programme™: www.icpkp.com

Chapter 20

DR. ROBERT SAMPSON
AND PATRICIA HUGHES

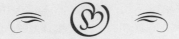

*T*hroughout this book, I have mentioned Dr. Robert Sampson and Patricia Hughes. Now I would like to focus on them, for they have been a huge influence on me and have taught me deep truths that have changed my understanding of life.

The day I met Robert, I came to him very tired and desperate. My life had become unbearable. My husband drove me, blindfolded. I was just a shell being led around—half alive.

Their office was located in a beautiful brick home. As I entered the residence, Robert greeted me gently. He recognized my state as fragile. He observed my old tattered gray outfit. Sitting across from him, I began my story. He listened kindly and smiled warmly. He had a beautiful smile! In a reassuring manner, he informed me that he, too, had also been ill with Environmental Illness. I felt I had finally arrived at the right doorstep and would find help with this gentle man.

He explained a little about his treatment plan, but I had no idea, that day, of the journey that would lie ahead of me if I followed the work of this brilliant man.

The first day, he carefully muscle tested me while he said many statements. I had no idea what was happening. I was so weak and tired of the whole illness that I just let him work. One time he had me turn around and he started to make a weird noise. I was thinking, "What have I gotten myself into?" when I felt a huge shift happen throughout my body. All of a sudden I stopped doubting and started to listen to him. He said he had balanced a chakra. At that time, the word *chakra* was new to me and meant nothing. I just felt it.

He worked seriously on me for about half an hour. Then he began my Nambudripad Allergy Elimination Treatment (NAET™). After muscle testing the first twelve substances Dr. Nambudripad has outlined, it was revealed that I required a treatment for sugar. When Dr. Sampson had finished massaging the back points, it was time for me to meet Patricia, who would complete the treatment.

Patricia was a petite, extremely pretty person. She came over to me with a beaming smile and laughed readily at something that was said. I liked her immediately. How pleasant she was! Yet beyond that pleasant exterior, she radiated a special healing quality that would inspire me and change me during the following months.

Patricia played a unique role in that office. Although on the surface she came in to massage the gate points, she played a much greater part. Her gentle, very intelligent words were deep with meaning and wisdom. She understood so much about truth and the universe. She imparted ideas that filled me with wonder. She also had the uncanny ability to know when I was ready to expand my knowledge.

Never going too quickly, she challenged my mind ever so gently more and more.

Through her loving words of encouragement, I dared to hope that I might recover completely and be directed to an even more enriching life than prior to the injury. She spoke of Environmental Illness as a "transformational condition," as one where the soul reaches new understanding and enlightenment. So much to look forward to! How could I see this terrible time as one of promise and freedom? Patricia's words were new and sometimes jarring, but oh, they were so beautiful and cherished!

Just before I had come to these fine healers, I had thought that Environmental Illness was a physical problem only. I knew that something was injured in my body during the exposure. None of the treatments from any of the doctors could penetrate the illness. I was beginning to realize that this injury could be more than just physical. My horizons were expanding and I was at the doorstep to a whole new understanding. When I met Robert and Patricia, I had just signed up for my doctorate at the American Institute of Hypnotherapy. I had prayed every day to the Blessed Mother and it seemed as though answers were coming to me and I was starting to listen. I know deep within that I had not happened upon these great healers by "accident." They had been clearly indicated to me and I had complied.

Even the circumstances leading me to them were clearly divinely inspired. I had spoken to Patricia on a Monday, for she had come to the support group with Robert to speak, and I had heard of them from my telephone friends. When Patricia and I conversed, I had a difficult time comprehending what she was talking about, for she spoke about "energetic healing." This meant nothing to me at that time.

The next day, Tuesday, I had prayed on the phone with a person on Father McDonough's prayer line. The following day, Doctor Dyler in Oregon, with whom I was consulting about herbs, told me about the new and exciting treatment NAET™ that eliminates allergies! He encouraged me to call Dr. Nambudripad to receive the list of treating practitioners in my area. When I called California for this list, I was surprised to see Dr Sampson and Patricia Hughes on it! By Friday of that same week, I was in their office.

There was no question that I was being led to them. I only wondered how I would ever understand them. They seemed to speak a foreign language initially. Words such as *chakra, energetic level, muscle testing, energy balancing,* and many other phrases were completely new. It took several months for me to grasp what they were saying and how to apply this knowledge to my healing.

Together, Robert and Patricia have co-authored a book entitled, *Breaking Out of Environmental Illness.* In the book, they relate their experiences with sensitivities and their struggles with the illness. They eventually decide that they should be together in life and join their talents to resolve their problems. Locating appropriate living conditions posed a great deal of difficulty for them. Their journey through the events is very sad and heartrending.

As I read the book, I could relate so well to their trials and efforts just to survive safely.

In the last section, they share their methods for healing and the treatments that helped them recover. Basically, they discuss the need to change their beliefs surrounding their illness. They also examine their reluctance to be totally present on the earth. As they alter their beliefs and observe their reactions from a more objective point of view, they begin their healing journey.

Their book contains some profound wisdom. It is important to be ready for very new and stirring ideas.

In my treatment sessions, I gained from the lessons they had learned during their illnesses. Their insight into Environmental Illness was significant. The energy work I received from Robert was excellent, but his wisdom and observations were equally valuable.

In their care, I believe that I received far more than NAET™ treatments. I began to realize that I was very fearful of the world and that, indeed, I did not really want to be totally present on this earth. I did not know if that was the case before my injury, but I surely knew it was so during the illness. The sicker I became, the more frightened I became. I perceived the world as dangerous and harmful to me. Gently and carefully, Robert and Patricia showed me that the world was whatever I saw it to be. As I gradually became stronger, I grew less and less afraid.

Patricia instructed me to watch what limiting statements I was giving to myself. One time we were having a light discussion about a vacation wherein she had enjoyed swimming in the hotel pool. I became discouraged and immediately stated, "I'll never be able to do that again." Quietly and seriously, she paused and considered my remark. She pointed out that if I said that and believed that, then, indeed, I would never be able to do it again. She cautioned me about limiting myself—something I did frequently. After that session, I noticed when I would do it, and gradually, I stopped. Instead, I would say, "When I'm better, I'll be able to . . ." I kept the door open for anything in the future. I also noticed how many times my EI friends would restrict themselves. It was amazing. This illness leads a person to believe that he or she will never be free to enjoy life or be totally present on the earth again.

So, thanks to Patricia and Robert, I incorporated the following suggestion into my hypnosis, "I am totally present on this earth, and it feels wonderful."

Often, when issues would arise in my treatment session, I would reinforce their solutions in my hypnosis plan. I would structure the suggestions to fit the spiritual growth I was experiencing at the time. This would help integrate a new idea into my subconscious. The changes would be faster and my healing would reap the positive results.

Robert and Patricia constantly assisted me and made me aware of my thoughts and emotions, which gradually changed from frightened restrictive beliefs to open and hopeful new awarenesses. They were offering special gifts and I was gratefully receiving!

Initially, I was reluctant to accept their views and the level of their understanding. How could I be playing such a powerful role in my own illness? I realized that I was motivating and directing events far more than I had ever imagined. At times I felt frustrated and confused—it was so hard to understand why I would be so blocked and stuck! Later, I just stopped judging myself and accepted my role—I decided to guide myself to a more positive outcome! With the assistance of Robert and Patricia, I was finally grasping my own role in the condition. As soon as I began to comprehend this, and work with them, my health began to improve. I felt stronger and more stable. No longer did I feel like a victim, but rather like a participant in the process.

As I worked with them, much of their information became easier to assimilate. The vocabulary and the concepts were so logical—once I tuned into them.

There was still the idea of energy and health that I desired to understand better in order to incorporate it effectively into my healing plan.

Chapter 21

ENERGY—ENERGY—ENERGY!

*I*t was December of 1996. I continued to gain back many lost activities. The most precious was that of being able to dry myself and wrap up in a cotton towel after a shower. I was also able to take a longer shower, now that I was not allergic to the chemicals in the water. It was luxurious!

On Christmas Eve, I was able to be around my family members for a holiday dinner! They were all careful not to wear fragrances. Fortunately, that was all they had to do; before they had had to wear old clothes, not shampoo their hair before they came, plus many other specific requests. There had been many restrictions. And I still had difficulty being around my loved ones!

This Christmas Eve was a wonderful and hopeful one. I actually enjoyed my family. I wore a fairly decent outfit of old cotton. It wasn't my gray outfit! Although I still appeared weak, I was coming along. Things were looking up.

I could have no presents, for I could not be around anything new and I could not even tolerate the wrapping paper. There were no decorations in my home and no tree, but I was so happy that I was healing. I loved taking rides with David to look at the Christmas lights. We were both feeling a little relieved.

My eyes were somewhat stronger. I was finally able to watch television. I was limited to two hours a day, but that was plenty for me. We had to move the television into the room adjoining our den. It was in the sunroom with glass doors between the rooms. I had to watch through the glass doors so that I would not breathe the fumes from the television. My husband rigged up a speaker in the den and I was able to listen to the television with a soft volume. The world was opening up to me.

During this time, I read the book, *Say Goodbye To Illness,* by Dr. Devi Nambudripad a second time. She discussed energy meridians and blocked energy pathways. This blocking process appeared to be a central problem for a person who has allergies. So, I began working to incorporate this idea into my hypnosis sessions.

I figured out that if suggestions were phrased properly, the subconscious might be assisted in the process of eliminating allergies. Also, If I coordinated the suggestions with the idea behind an NAET™ treatment, then I could further help the clearing to be easier and more comfortable for my body!

This was accomplished by including suggestions about opening the energy meridians in the hypnosis session. Using this method, the innate intelligence of the body is given reinforcement to learn the pattern used in the NAET™ technique. This can accelerate the process of clearing sensitivities and strengthen the inner acceptance of it. Although I have used some of these "energy" suggestions earlier in this book, I will now explain their placement in the hypnosis script so that you may be clear about the proper use of these important suggestions for the elimination of allergies.

As you will observe below, the "Angel of Healing" section is very similar to the one contained in Chapter 17. There is no need to alter your script. The issue is discussed here to clarify why the suggestion concerning energy is very important and where it should be inserted in order to achieve optimum results.

In each section of the hypnosis script covered in this chapter, the suggestions concerning energy are written in bold print.

I am now going to a beautiful place to allow my body to be healed and renewed. It is a peaceful secluded ocean beach. The sky is blue and the white, fluffy clouds are drifting peacefully, and gently by. I feel a lovely warm breeze and my body feels wonderful. The air is crystal clear and as I breathe it, I fill my body with fresh, clean air. There are birds chirping softly in the distance. They are bringing me good luck and good fortune.

The Angel of Healing comes to this setting with her golden hands and golden fingers of healing. She gives me a golden robe to adorn my body for this special healing time. There is a lovely, soft, silky bed to lie upon and I prepare for this wonderful healing experience.

As the Angel of Healing touches each part of my body, the energy meridians to that part of the body are opened, bringing sufficient energy to that area so that it works perfectly for me. She brings health and strength to each area she touches.

My next step was to proceed to have the angel touch all the major organs gently and any part of my body that needed to heal or required extra attention. It was a very soothing and wonderful part, which I used each time. In Chapter 17, I have outlined this section.

As a quick review, please remember that it is not necessary to discuss the exact function precisely, for the organ knows its role within the body perfectly. For example, in healing the liver, one might say, "Ever so gently, the Angel Of Healing touches my liver. It detoxifies substances easily for me and performs all its functions perfectly for the good of my entire body."

I only mention detoxification because this is a focus for most EI people. Then I just add that it performs all its function perfectly. I do not advise that the exact functions be discussed. This might cause confusion if you are not exactly correct. Besides, the body knows precisely what it is supposed to do.

Later, during the end-result imagery, I again emphasize the issue of energy. I say that I picture myself perfectly healthy, doing whatever I wish to do. I make certain that the scene becomes very clear. Then I make some very positive statements about how I feel when I am completely healthy. The important statement concerning energy is as follows:

My energy meridians remain open when other energy fields come in contact with mine. It feels wonderful to be open and clear.

This again encourages the subconscious to open the energy meridians along with what is being accomplished manually with the NAET™ treatments.

Then for a third time, at the last stage of the session, once again I suggest:

My energy meridians remain open when other energy fields come in contact with mine, and it feels wonderful to be strong and open.

In this manner, I have repeated in many ways, at different stages of the session, that I wish for my energy meridians to remain open when I am in contact with the energies of other substances. This is a clear message for my subconscious.

This is a very nice way to reinforce the NAET™ treatments and to encourage the body to heal itself. Many times the allergies can clear themselves when the body becomes accustomed to opening. The body's innate intelligence may begin to take over the work, and a new pattern becomes established. It is very desirable to encourage the subconscious to learn the process and to clear automatically. Fewer NAET™ treatments will be required once the body acquires the ability to eliminate allergies all by itself!

In my case, I began to be able to clear allergies at home using the gate points only. Because I was able to muscle test myself, I could verify that I had cleared an allergy 100 percent. Also, when I would see Dr. Sampson to be given other "official" treatments, he would find that I had cleared several of the substances to which I had previously tested "sensitive." I no longer required a treatment for them. Dr. Sampson admitted that he observed this in other patients to some degree, but not to the extent that he saw it in my case. I attribute this to my attention paid to this issue in my hypnosis sessions.

Often, in the early stages of Environmental Illness, many people experience the phenomenon of "spreading," which is the addition of more and more allergies. This is a closing pattern and the body becomes more and more blocked. Now, through the suggestions in hypnosis, the body receives a new message, that it is time to open the energy meridians and clear the body of allergies.

The winter was a long one for me, but my efforts were centered on clearing my allergies and preparing for the lovely spring that was soon approaching.

Chapter 22

FLOWERS!

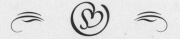

*T*hat winter of 1997 had ended and it had blossomed into a delightful and warm spring. I still could not go outside, due to the light sensitivity. This was very frustrating and disappointing to me. From my kitchen window, I watched my neighbors plant their flowers. I used to have beautiful flower gardens. Observing the different flowers bloom as spring progressed filled me with wonder and joy. I had attended lovingly to the various plantings for years so that they were quite well-established. The perennial flowers continued to bloom. David tried to maintain them for me; he knew how much I cherished my gardens. This was difficult for him, because he was still working day and night to earn enough money so that we would not lose our house. Finances were tight and I worried all the time. I had lost my entire salary and it was hard for David. He tried not to complain, but I rarely saw him due to the extra hours he had to put in.

One day I heard some noise on the front doorstep. When I opened the door, I saw no one. However, on the step was a beautiful cutting of fresh flowers. I was so touched. I knew it was from one of my wonderful neighbors. They knew how much I loved flowers and that I could not tend to mine. I never found out who put them there, but I cherished the moment of knowing someone cared. Naturally, I could not keep them inside, so I put them in a vase and put them outside my window. What a special gift!

As always, the happy moments were interspersed with times of great challenge and disappointment. Soon, I would be facing another roadblock, and my fortitude would be tested yet again!

Chapter 23

MORE BAD NEWS

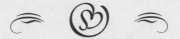

*T*hat spring, I was summoned to the Retirement Board meeting. The members had received all the reports from their three doctors. My lawyer accompanied me. The Commissioner of Education for Massachusetts was the chairman of this board. He directed his questions at me. He didn't allow my lawyer to contribute much at all. I related my sad story about my injury. My intention was to be entirely truthful and sincere. My voice was weak but firm as I clearly detailed the order of events and the resulting destruction of my life. The board regarded me quietly. I did my best to convey the misery of my life and the total lack of ability to live it as I was once able to.

Immediately upon the conclusion of his brief questions, he promptly announced that they just did not have enough information to grant me a pension. Before the board, on the table, was a bulging folder of information concerning my case and that was not enough! I was dismayed. Yet another attempt to not help me!

The commissioner continued and announced that they would pose more questions to the doctors. He would notify us when he received the answers. So, I went home with nothing again! The legal bills were mounting sharply and I was being denied any assistance.

As everyone stood up to leave, I realized that I could not muster enough strength to get out of my chair. My legs would not carry me. So much of my strength had been used to convey my story and to come into Boston. One man saw my struggle and assisted me until I could stand up. My life was crumbling and now I felt the weight of all this strain.

The reality of my bleak situation felt heavy on the ride home. My injury was one they could not understand. I did not truly understand it either, but it was real and it was disabling! Why was it all so difficult!

After three months, I was summoned again by the board. Their original three doctors had been firm in their opinions. Two reiterated their position that I had been harmed by the roofing fumes. The third, (the anesthesiologist) had agreed that I was totally disabled, but was not sure why. A vote of two out of three was required to grant a pension.

Deep inside, I was hoping that this second meeting would suffice to receive my pension. What more could they do to block it? Their own doctors insisted that I should be compensated. I was so tired of this terrible treatment just because I had MCS. I was not prepared for what would ensue at this absurd meeting.

My attorney and I were taken completely by surprise when the commissioner announced that the board had held a "private" meeting with yet another doctor—one who had never met or examined me. The commissioner explained that this doctor attended the "private" meeting to discuss MCS. My lawyer and I weren't invited. Based on this secret meeting, I was refused my pension! The commissioner said that this new doctor agreed that MCS is a controversial illness.

Since that concurred with the board's opinion, they were firm in their denial!

My attorney was astonished. They had denied my "right to an open meeting." As we departed the room, she exclaimed to me that she had never seen anything as outrageous as the treatment they issued to me. Why were they so adamant in their refusal to acknowledge MCS? Could it be that there were so may other cases waiting in the wings to be considered? If I won, would that set a precedent that would allow a landslide of similar cases? Whatever the reason, I was defeated!

I do not understand why they spent months and months of my time sending me to doctors only to refuse me because they did not understand MCS. Isn't that what the panel of doctors was for? I was so weary of this unfair treatment. I felt horrible. I just could not win! There were two other teachers there that day with Environmental Illnesses and they, too, were refused. The only difference with them was that they belonged to a different union and their union was picking up the tab. My union had refused to help me even though I had tried several times to ask them for assistance. I even asked them to pay only some of my legal fees. They kept insisting that my union only paid for a teacher if he or she were accused of wrongdoing. They said they could not afford to help teachers who were injured at work.

The other two women assumed they would appeal. I had yet another decision to make. Could I appeal? I already owed several thousand dollars in trying to get my pension. Now it would mean several thousand more. It seemed like a no-win situation.

I am relating these events to explain that Environmental Illness has many problems attached to it. Not only might you lose your career and your life as you've known it, but you may also have a very difficult time proving that you have an illness and receiving your much-deserved benefits. Researchers have not developed a test for it yet, so you are vulnerable to the doubts and disbelief of the public and the medical profession.

Doctors and researchers must work conscientiously to acknowledge this very real problem and to validate this illness. People should not be left penniless just because they tried to perform their jobs in an unhealthy environment and got injured. Perhaps if the employers are made responsible for their employees' health, they will be much more careful about what they expose their workers to. Many cases of Environmental Illness can be avoided. It is such a shame to lose your life or years from your life because of careless employers.

Now I had a decision to make and another wound to heal. However, I was on a healing trend and I was determined not to let these disappointments stand in my way!

Chapter 24

REFRAMING

I worked on letting go of my anger about these losses so that it would not block me from healing. I kept my mind busy studying hypnosis and writing my papers. Each week I went to Robert and Patricia and I did hypnosis once a week as well. I had a job to do and I was intent on doing it!

During my hypnosis studies, I read a book entitled, *My Voice Will Go With You,* by Sidney Rosen, about an interesting man named Milton Erickson, who was a very famous hypnotherapist. He lived in Arizona. What was truly amazing about him was that he had had polio as a young child and could not move his body. He could only move his eyes. By watching the people around him, he became a master of observation.

He used self-hypnosis and gradually regained the use of his arms and legs. However, he spent most of his time in a wheelchair. He used hypnosis every morning to alleviate the pain and he completed the remainder of his day comfortably.

He learned how to observe his clients and to establish a rapport with them. He was able to reach deep into the subconscious and achieve remarkable results. One of his methods was to use teaching tales. The individual would think he was listening to a story, but really Erickson was talking to the subconscious mind and altering the way the person viewed a problem.

Erickson often helped his client to see his problem in a new light, and in doing so, the person came away with an understanding that it was not so terrible. He might even interpret the problem as a blessing in some way. Erickson called this *reframing*. The author, Sidney Rosen, also talks about this when he refers to Victor Frankl's time in a concentration camp:

> While most of his fellow inmates lost hope and subsequently died, Frankl occupied his mind thinking about the lectures he would give after his release— lectures that would draw on his experience in the camp. Thus, he reframed the potentially deadening and hopeless situation. He transformed it in his mind to a source of rich experiences that he could use to help others overcome apparently hopeless situations—physical or mental.[1]

Suddenly, I realized that I was doing just this kind of thing. As I studied and learned, I was accomplishing something special with this time of my life. Instead of it being simply a time to suffer and be angry and disappointed at the school, the legal system, and some members of the medical profession, I was learning about health and the mind. I was acquiring a doctorate. Perhaps, I would be able to look back at

---

[1] **Chapter 24:** Sidney Rosen, *My Voice Will Go With You: The Teaching Tales of Milton Erickson* (New York, NY: W.W. Norton & Company, 1991), 143.

this potentially lonely and dismal time and see it as an enriching time, during which I greatly expanded my mind and spirit. I certainly hoped so!

PART IV

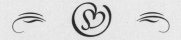

The bridge is built. It is of gold. I now must cross as the Blessed Mother guides me. I am cautious, for I do not know what awaits me on the other side.

Chapter 25

CONGRATULATIONS, DOCTOR SMITH!

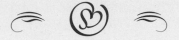

*A*s the summer of 1997 approached, I was nearing the completion of my hypnosis studies. Enriching my mind about the inner abilities of healing had been a wonderful experience. Great attention was being paid to my mind and my beliefs. I realized that in order to heal this very serious injury, I needed to call upon *all* my resources. I worked diligently on giving my subconscious mind clear pictures and direction for where I wanted to go, that is, to heal completely. This work centered around my mental and emotional levels. These layers were also addressed during my sessions with Patricia.

In addition to the mental and emotional levels, there are three other levels that need to be addressed in order to recover from an illness of this magnitude. These levels include the energetic level, the spiritual level, and of course, the physical level.

I worked each week on my energetic body, making sure that the energy flow was becoming clearer and clearer throughout my body. This was accomplished by my NAET™ treatments and the "100 percent willing" work with Dr. Sampson and Patricia. Also, clearing traumas with the TAT™ method was opening the energy pathways.

The spiritual level was very important—I grew closer and closer to the dear Blessed Mother. Each day, I prayed a rosary to her and asked her to lead me out of this illness. My sensitivity had reached the rosary beads as well. When I handled them, I reacted, so I had to count out the appropriate number of "Hail Marys" and just repeat the prayer. Her presence was so calming in the midst of this turmoil. One day I asked her to guide me to serve a purpose on this earth. I prayed, "Please don't let me be wasted in this room for the rest of my life." I offered my assistance to her in any way she saw fit. This was a serious moment for me and I remember feeling filled with her love as I made this agreement from the depths of my soul. Time would tell how she would decide to direct me.

Now I needed to focus carefully on the physical level. My knowledge of herbs and vitamins was rapidly growing. I used some and obtained great benefit from them; however, if I were going to totally heal myself, I needed a much better understanding of how the body works and what can truly strengthen and rebuild it.

I began researching quality programs to locate one that would complete my knowledge. One friend suggested Trinity College of Natural Health in Indiana. I inquired there and was pleased with what I was told.

They offered a course of study about a variety of subjects, which included some I had not known much about, such as iridology and foot reflexology. Iridology is the study of the iris of the eye, made well-known during this century by a man named

Dr. Bernard Jensen. His contention is that each area of the iris in the eye corresponds with an area of the body; information can be obtained about the general condition of every part of the body. The healing process can also be reflected by changes within the iris—thus the name "iridology." Reflexology is the usage of acupressure points on the bottom and sides of the foot to bring about better health within the body. These two areas of study had always intrigued me.

The strongest emphasis of learning was on nutrition and healing—just what I was looking for! There was also a heavy concentration on herbology, the use of herbs in healing—another of my favorite subjects. I was becoming interested.

That evening, I discussed with David my desire to become a naturopath, the degree awarded by this school. He was surprised. He reminded me that I had not even finished my hypnosis studies and that that was already a very heavy amount of work. He was concerned that I might be taking on too much and might endanger my health. I assured him I could do it, and by the time the registration was processed and new material arrived, I would have completed my AIH studies. He laughed; he saw that there was no reasoning with me. He agreed to pay for this school. We hadn't even finished paying for The American Institute of Hypnotherapy yet! Poor David. I asked so much of him, however, I needed to get well so that I could be a contributing member of our family in the ways that I had before my injury. We both realized that if there were no answers to this illness from the medical community, I would have to seek them myself.

So, I signed up!

Over the summer, I intensified my efforts to complete my work for AIH. I was almost sad that it was nearing completion. It had been my light during a very dark time. I would have been so lost and lonely without it. This focus had given me hope and direction. Each day, as I read the pages containing positive words of encouragement, empowerment, and determination, I grew more and more certain that the healing gift was within my own grasp. My only requirement was to engage the inner abilities of healing that were so readily available to me.

By this time, I was able to type the long involved papers myself on the computer. David had only needed to type the first eight! After that, I took over. I had gained the ability to use the computer for fifteen minutes in the morning and fifteen minutes in the evening. That was enough for me to accomplish the task. I would write out the papers by hand (eight hundred pages in all) and then, very quickly, type them out on the computer. I continued to read all the material and books through my glass dining-room table. This was tiring to my body, but wonderful for my mind. All my energy and attention was focused on the idea of healing, not on being sick.

As August approached, it was time for my final oral exam. Dr. Neves, my advisor, scheduled the date. I had two weeks to prepare. I reviewed all the concepts I had learned and I read over my papers. There was so much material! I had no idea what he would ask me. Dr. Neves was such a very intelligent man. Along with his role as a director at AIH, he was also a hypnotherapist. He knew his craft well. During my studies, whenever I had a question, he answered it insightfully. He explained things clearly in his wonderfully rich voice—I could easily imagine how well he must have been able to "put people under."

I was quite confident that I would perform well, for I had thoroughly enjoyed the knowledge imparted by the studies. However, one thing was worrying me. I had always had difficulty hearing Dr. Neves because he used a headset and I had a speaker-phone. At times, he would turn away from the headset and his voice would become inaudible. I had never mentioned this, for it was not crucial to hear every word before. Now I knew that I must deal with this issue, for I might answer incorrectly if I could not hear the question properly. I was reluctant to inform him that I was injured. I did not want him to think less of me. Perhaps this was a bad attitude, but I didn't think a lot of myself after this injury. My self-esteem was very low. I had never wanted to ask for special treatment. My desire was to do all the work and receive my degree just like anybody else.

Finally, the day arrived. This was it! Dr. Neves called me and we began. I confided in him that I was using a speaker-phone because of an impairment and therefore, he needed to speak into his headset directly so that I could hear him. He expressed surprise. He was very understanding. To console and comfort me, he confided that he, too, had overcome a serious medical condition using hypnosis. He encouraged me and gave me a wonderful feeling of knowing that I could indeed heal completely and that my work was excellent. I should have informed him of my plight sooner!

The exam went smoothly and I soon calmed down. He asked me about all the required reading. We discussed various hypnotic techniques and the work of many hypnotherapists, including Milton Erickson, Dr. Krasner, and Carl and Stephanie Simonton. There were many texts and the discussion moved quickly from one to the other. Responding to each question was easy for me; my life had centered around these works and they had inspired me so.

After being satisfied that I had grasped the concepts fully, he moved on to the elective texts. Some of the books I had chosen dealt with Neuro Linguistic Programming (NLP), hypnosis with children, and the study of past lives—a topic that had intrigued me for many years. We conversed for an hour and a half. We discussed many of the concepts contained in the reading. I had no difficulty, for it had been my whole life. I passed the exam!

Then, in his resonant voice, Dr. Neves announced, "Congratulations, Dr. Smith." I was elated. It had really happened. I had climbed the mountain!

I called David and he was thrilled. Something good had finally happened to us. He was as happy as I was. That week he surprised me with a little cake. On the top, the words read, "Congratulations, Dr. Smith!"

Chapter 26

THE SOUND OF MUSIC

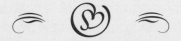

*T*hat September, the fall of 1997, marked three years since my injury. I think this was the worst September for me. I was stronger and healing so I wanted very much to be back at school. I missed it so much that I dreamed of it every morning just before awakening. My repetitive dream was that I was in the school hiding out and teaching. I didn't want anyone to find me and make me leave. Then, every time, someone found me, usually an administrator, and led me out of the school. I was left in the parking lot looking back at the school, alone and sad.

When I awoke from these dreams, I was crushed. The reality of my situation would hit me and I would feel so alone. I would feel like such a failure. Why had this happened to me? Then I would convince myself to get up and face the day. I knew in my heart and mind that my teaching career was over and that I could not ever consider going back, for I was far too ill.

That fall was so sad and lonely. However, one day something special and lovely happened. I was walking by the living room, which I could not be in for more than ten minutes. My piano was covered, as it had been for three years now. My ears were hurt too much to hear any piano music. I decided to give it a try.

I opened the piano and regarded the beckoning white and black ivories. How long it had been! Hesitantly, I began to play. For some reason, I selected musicals and, one after another, they resonated through the living room. *Camelot* was first, then *Sound of Music, Fiddler on the Roof,* and finally, *Cinderella.* Such lovely *lovely* songs! The music sounded wonderful and felt pleasant to my ears—as it used to before so much had gone wrong! I was deeply moved. For about twenty minutes, I was able to listen to music and be in the living room without difficulty! I had music back! Even if only for a short time, I had my music back! I played softly and smoothly. It was as if I had never stopped playing. The music came and the songs were beautiful. My hands were quick and strong. Years and years of playing had trained me and now I was playing the piano again.

This was yet another piece of me, now replaced— music for me isn't a hobby, it is a part of my soul. I felt like Humpty Dumpty with all the missing pieces. I wondered if "all the king's horses and all the king's men" could put me back together again! I was so broken. But now there was some hope. Maybe someday I would be able to listen to music for a long time and truly enjoy it again. At least I had hope.

Chapter 27

GET DRESSED!

*E*ven though my health was improving, my spirits were very low. I was sad all the time. The reality of my lost career was hitting me and I could not be consoled. I had taught for twenty years—humanities, social studies, French, German, Spanish, and history. I had loved every subject. My students perceived that I truly cared about them and I was considered to be an excellent teacher. The children always came to me when they had problems. I guess they understood that I was the approachable one. I wanted them to learn and to enjoy the wonders of learning. As I strove to enrich each lesson, I tried to make it meaningful for them. Along with the academics, I taught them about goodness and kindness toward one another. I always believed that teachers are more then just educators. We are role models. Children learn from observing us as well as listening to us.

Now all that was over. I felt alone and useless. I was listless, and when I went for my treatments to Robert, he noticed my down attitude. He was working alone, because Patricia was taking a break and working fewer days.

One day, without much enthusiasm, I asked him if I could assist him, since Patricia was not there. He was surprised, but he did not say no. I thought that he would, because I felt that no one would want me now.

The next time I arrived for my appointment, Robert surprised me as he cleared his throat and began, "Patricia and I would be delighted to include you here as a practitioner. However, rather than working for me, why don't you begin your own practice as a hypnotherapist? You may rent one of my treatment rooms where you will be safe to work."

I was speechless and surprised. Patricia was present that day and she noticed my fear and reluctance. I sat and listened as she encouraged me. She coaxed, "Just begin at a very slow pace and you will be helping others who are very sick—as you once were. It's time to begin your new life."

I was very nervous with this conversation. I felt so confused. I didn't know who I was anymore. My identity was changing and I was not sure I could adjust. I had always thought of myself as a teacher. Now I was a doctor of hypnotherapy. Could I really help others?

After our discussion, I replied, "I'll consider your idea. I just have to think about it for awhile."

They were so helpful to me and so kind. I guess they understood my predicament—they too had been there. Perhaps another doctor had helped them get started again.

While pondering their suggestion, I found that I was indeed happy to think of being useful again. I was even more pleased and honored that they would want me around them, for I felt so undesirable as a person. I knew I needed to work on this attitude, but I think it results from this illness. I hoped that in time my feeling of self-worth would improve.

After some deliberation, I decided that I would like to begin treating others using hypnosis. However, a huge block still existed. I had only two outfits I could wear. Clothes were still a major problem for me. I had the now worn-to-a-frazzle gray outfit and one other pair of pants and a sweater. They just were too old and worn-out for a professional person or for anyone. How could I help others believe in me if I could not even wear clothes? So, now I would focus all my attention on getting my clothes back.

To achieve this objective, I incorporated suggestions about clothes in my hypnosis session. I began repeating the suggestions throughout the session. In the end-result imagery portion, I visualized myself wearing whatever I wanted. In a later part of the session, I stated, "I can wear clothes easily and it feels wonderful to be able to wear clothes."

By focusing on this issue in hypnosis, I was attempting to remove the fear about venturing into this new area of sensitivities. If I could remain in a deeply relaxed state while mentioning wearing clothes, I could perhaps coax my inner self to feel calm about the prospect of donning attractive outfits once again.

My two closets of clothes posed a problem for me—they had perfume and scents on them. Before I was injured, I could use perfume and I did— liberally! Also, the clothing was made of a variety of fabrics. Previously, it never mattered what I wore. If I liked the texture, color, and fit, I purchased it. I never had to worry about anything, for I was not at all sensitive.

Since my injury, I decided to build a wardrobe of cotton clothing—I really didn't have much that was "all cotton." I had always steered away from cotton— for I thought it shrank and wrinkled too much.

David had bought me four cotton cardigans from Lands' End, a catalog clothing company, the year before. I had protested that I could not wear them. He had insisted that someday I would need them and when I was ready, they would be ready for me. We had hung them in the loft to air out. David was so thoughtful and so optimistic!

This day, I needed them, and so, I went out to the loft. The four garments were hanging there just waiting for me. I walked over to them. I had not really looked at them before—I was too sad and discouraged about clothes. Looking carefully at the beautiful colors, I wondered if I would really be able to wear these lovely clothes. They were light blue, coral, pink, and green—very pretty, vibrant colors. I had only worn gray and navy-blue for years. How would it feel to wear these bright colors? I was nervous. I slowly took the pink one down and tried it on. It fit perfectly. I started to react when I held it in my hand. How would I ever be able to wear it? By this point, I had learned to clear allergies at home—after using the NAET™ treatments long enough, your body can clear substances very easily. So, now I began to use gate points to clear it. I massaged the points the number of times my body had indicated through muscle testing. Then I waited two days to let the treatment process.

For two days, I kept peeking at the soft fabric of these clothes hanging in the loft. Excitement was building. The four cardigans held the key that would release me from of the prison of Environmental Illness. Once I could wear them, I could make my way into the world as a doctor and begin a new life! I also checked about being "100 percent willing" to wear clothes, and to go back out into the world. So much was riding on placing this new apparel on my body!

Finally, after the two days of processing, I ventured into the loft to try on the lovely pink cardigan. It was fine. I didn't react! I could wear it! I also had selected a cream-colored pair of slacks and a cream jersey—also made of cotton— from my closet; they were fine for me. I wore them under the cardigan and voilà! I had a very nice looking outfit. I looked like a real doctor!

The next week, I surprised Robert and Patricia as I walked in wearing the outfit. They were ecstatic for me. They had given me the motivation to work on wearing clothes and I was on my way. I didn't start working with clients at that time, but I was getting ready and my spirits were lifting.

Once again Robert and Patricia had helped me. They were encouraging me to move forward at a safe pace, and I so needed to do that. Maybe I could actually have a life again.

Thank you, Robert and Patricia—and *Lorri!*

Chapter 28

PHYSICAL HEALING

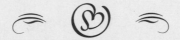

*L*ater that fall, my telephone friend Kathy sensed my sadness about my lost career and the poor treatment from the legal system. She strongly suggested I see her psychologist, Dr. Weiser. I was hesitant. I didn't see how he could help. Reluctantly, I called him and he seemed very understanding. So I made an appointment.

The first visit was difficult. I cried and had great difficulty talking about the injury. It was just so painful. I saw him for a few weeks. He kept asking me to talk about the struggles I was going through. I didn't like this and felt that it was hard enough to live with MCS, without having to dwell on it. He saw my reluctance.

One week, he asked me to talk about my past, before the injury. I began slowly, because it was actually difficult to remember the time before. Then I gradually slipped into this peaceful reminiscent state. "Before this happened to me, I loved to ski and play tennis. My deep connection for the mountains led me to sign up for a year in Switzerland my junior year at college. How spiritual I felt skiing serenely down the majestic Alps. Only a magnificent God could create these slopes."

Dr. Weiser was smiling. He, too, had studied in Switzerland and he now also slipped into pleasant reverie. I felt more and more alive as I continued discussing my past. "Often I think of my students. What joy they gave me! Their young trusting faces smiling as they learned new wonders. Sometimes they laughed with me when a funny event happened in our classroom. Laughter is so wonderful for the bond between humans. Children often left my classroom so much lighter and more peaceful than they entered." As I reviewed the highlights of my once fulfilling life, I remembered the person who loved music, flowers, children, and beautiful sunny days at the ocean.

I realized after that appointment that the happy person was still inside and I had not completely lost her. I just needed to clear enough of the pain and sorrow so that she might have a chance to live again. That was the great gift Dr. Weiser gave to me. I didn't need to see him very much after that. He had done something wonderful. He had helped me to open up and find myself. I remembered that I was a good person who deserved to heal and smile again.

Also, during that fall, I was heavily involved with my naturopathic studies. I was learning a great deal about the body and how it worked. Book after book arrived and I read for hours and hours each day. Although I learned about many theories and treatments, there were two authors who imparted the most valuable information to me: Dr. M. Ted Morter Jr. and Dr. Bernard Jensen. I would like to share their ideas about nutrition with you.

First, I found Dr. M. Ted Morter Jr. to be very interesting. He authored a book entitled, *Your Health . . . Your Choice.* In this work, he talks about how to maintain health in the body. He first discusses his theory of disease. He attributes it to three main causes. They are TOXICITY, TIMING, and THOUGHTS.

When he speaks of TOXICITY, he refers to having too much acid in the body. This can occur from eating excessive amounts of *acid* ash-producing foods. They include protein foods such as meat, fish, and poultry. Also, grains produce acid, but to a lesser degree.

Dr. Morter also explains that improper internal TIMING happens when one of our natural physiological functions occurs at an inappropriate time. For example, it is correct for the muscles to become tense before a physical activity. However, it is not correct to tense up while on his examining table. This is improper internal timing. He explains that this happens because:

> The body responds to stimuli from a database (memory bank), that is programmed for survival at the moment. Pain and health problems arise when your body responds to stimuli from past conditions that no longer exist—obsolete programming.[1]

Dr. Morter believes that suggestions to the subconscious can be helpful in these situations. If a person experiences pain months after an accident or event, for no apparent reason, and his muscles remain tense, he needs to stop the connection from his data bank. The subconscious can help break this improper physiological response.

The third cause of disease is THOUGHTS—he explains that your body experiences as strong an emotional reaction to a *perceived* threat as it does to the

---

[1] **Chapter 28:** Dr. Ted Morter Jr., *Your Health. . . Your Choice* (Hollywood, FL: Lifetime Books, Inc. 1995), 28.

actual event. These negative thoughts produce more acid in your body than anything else.

He suggests that a problem with any one of these three principles, TOXICITY, TIMING, or THOUGHTS, can result in fatigue, a lowered immune system, and finally illness.[2]

His text deals primarily with the concept that an acidic body is a toxic one. He encourages the reader to eat more *alkaline* ash-producing foods. These are mostly vegetables and fruits. He advises the reader to limit his intake of protein foods that produce acid ash, such as meats, poultry, fish, and grains. His diet would ideally consist of the following:

45% cooked fruits and vegetables
30% raw fruits and vegetables
25% grains, nuts, seeds, meat, fish, or poultry

Using this model, he suggests that the reader gradually modify his diet to strengthen the alkaline reserves in the body. This leads to less toxicity and greater overall health.[3]

I read this text with much interest, for I had heard from many of my friends and doctors that allergies often render a person's body very acidic. I do not know if this is cause or effect. Perhaps a person becomes very allergic because he has eaten a diet of excessive protein and has become too acidic.

This research prompted me to monitor my diet. I saw that I did not eat enough raw foods. So, I added

[2] Ibid. pp. 25-30.
[3] Ibid. p. 231.

a salad four more times a week. Celery was also included to restore the natural sodium to my body. I made certain that I ate more vegetables and I added another fruit to my daily regimen.

I was careful not to eat too much fruit, for I did not want too much sugar in my system. There is the possibility of candida overgrowth for people who have weakened immune systems. I had had difficulty with candida during the beginning of my illness, and now I wanted to be careful to keep it under control.

Let me take a moment to explain how candida can play a role in an illness dealing with allergies. Candida (*candida albicans*) is a normal yeast that inhabits the intestinal tract. When immune problems arise, it can overgrow. Then it changes into the fungal form and can permeate the intestinal tract. This can cause small openings in the tract that permit food particles to go out into the blood stream, thus, making it much easier to form allergies to the foods. People with excessive candida may experience many food allergies. If this is suspected, measures can be taken, such as taking a type of intestinal flora known as acidophilus. This can help restore the balance of probiotic bacteria in the intestinal tract.

Also, sugar feeds candida and so it should be totally eliminated from the diet. There are many ways to help restore the intestinal balance. There are many books on this subject. If a careful diet is followed, the problem can be completely controlled.

One way many people develop problems with yeast is the overuse of antibiotics. Antibiotics destroy the beneficial intestinal flora as well as the bacteria they were intended to kill. Thus, if the "good" bacteria aren't reestablished in the gut, many health problems can result.

I am discussing candida, because this is a problem that should be addressed first if a person is very allergic; candida can be responsible for many food, pollen, and chemical allergies. Controlling and reducing the overgrowth of candida can make a wonderful improvement in your health. At the very least, it is important to rule the possibility of this contributing factor out.

There are some fine texts that deal exclusively with candida and how to control it. Two of them are listed in the appendix. Again, may I emphasize that this is a very serious issue to consider if you are dealing with many food allergies. Correcting this problem can make a noticeable difference in your health and greatly reduce your food intolerances.

A last issue, which I found to be very interesting in Dr. Morter's book, was that of food combining. I have read this idea in other texts and so I figured that perhaps it might be advisable to consider this information.

I have simplified his long list of rules. The basic idea is as follows:

- Fruit should be eaten alone and best if eaten in the morning. If possible, wait one hour before eating other food.
- Protein and starches require different digestive mediums and should not be combined in the same meal. (Good-bye steak and potatoes!)
- Protein and sugar is an unhealthy combination. (Au revoir ice cream!)
- Starches and fruits do not combine well. (Adios apple pie!)
- Vegetables can be eaten with protein.
- Vegetables can be eaten with starch.

• Liquids interfere with digestive fluids. They should not accompany a meal.[4]

Anthony Robbins writes of similar research in his book entitled, *Unlimited Power.* He states that eating protein with a starch interferes with, and even blocks, digestion. He goes on to explain that starchy foods (rice, bread, potatoes) require an alkaline environment, while protein foods (meat, dairy, nuts) require an acid environment. Two opposite mediums cannot work together because they neutralize one another. Foods become poorly digested and bacterial growth is promoted, causing fermentation. Discomfort and gas may result, as well as a depletion of energy.[5]

After reading this same idea from more than one source, I decided to learn from it. The main thing I had to stop was my favorite meat and potatoes combination. Now I realized it was probably not good for me for two reasons. First, there was the issue of too much protein, rendering me too acidic. Second, there was the improper combination of a protein and a starch.

These rules are guidelines to follow, but I did not feel the need to be obsessive about them. Whenever possible, I altered my food combinations to assist the digestive process. At other times, I allowed myself the enjoyment of some meat and potatoes, and once in a great while, some ice cream. I think moderation is a comfortable approach and can render positive results. The only rule I followed very seriously was NO SUGAR when I was healing a candida overgrowth!

[4] Ibid. p. 225

[5] Anthony Robbins, *Unlimited Power* (New York, NY: Ballantine Books, 1987), 175-176.

From that point forward, I have never reinstated a regular use of sugar in my diet.

There was so much to learn!

The next author I was very impressed with was Dr. Bernard Jensen. He seemed to possess a vast and comprehensive plan for restoring and retaining the health.

He authored *The Chemistry Of Man*. This comprehensive text deals with the chemical balance within the body. If the mineral balance is thrown off, many serious health problems can result. Dr. Jensen used nutrition to help restore the body's natural balance.

Many years ago, Dr. Jensen selected a beautiful site in Escondido, California and created his sanitarium called Hidden Valley Health Ranch. On the ranch, the patients grew much of their own vegetables and fruits. They kept their own chickens and goats for fresh eggs and milk.

His emphasis was toward getting and staying well.

He helped people recover by bringing them back to natural foods. He states that, "Only nature can come to our rescue. . . . In my view, the path to wholeness and high-level wellness starts with nutrition."[6]

He says there is one food we should absolutely avoid and that is sugar. He is also against coffee and chocolate. These are empty foods and can be harmful.

When he talks about sugar, he says, "White sugar processed from sugar cane or sugar beets is not merely neutral in its effect on the body, it is actually harmful." He lists many of the ways it can harm the body. Some include tooth decay, leaching calcium

---

[6] Bernard Jensen, Ph. D. *The Chemistry of Man* (Escondido, CA: Bernard, Jensen International, 1983), 17.

from the body so that it disturbs the delicate balance between calcium and phosphorus, and causing a deficiency of B vitamins.[7]

He further recommends avoiding processed foods and devitalized foods, such as white flour. He advises the reader to eat food that comes from the earth.

His dietary recommendation is to eat 80 percent alkaline foods (vegetables and fruits) and 20 percent acid foods (meat, fish, poultry, and grains). This concurs with Dr. Morter's idea as well.

Dr. Jensen does not recommend a vegetarian diet; he says that when he traveled to distant places, the people he saw who lived to be very old ate some meat.

His ideal daily diet consists of:

> Two different fruits, at least four to six vegetables, one protein, and one starch. Drink fruit and vegetable juices between meals. Eat at least two leafy green vegetables a day. Fifty to sixty percent of the foods you eat daily should be raw. Consider this regimen a dietary law.[8]

Now, I was armed with much more knowledge. I respected these two authors and they had a very logical approach to health. I could either be discouraged and think how aggravating to have to eat so many vegetables, or I could be pleased that there was yet another way I could heal my body. At first I was reluctant to begin the quest for four to six vegetables a day. Soon, however, I found it easy to accomplish this. Gradually, I realized that it was great to have this knowledge, which gave me more control over my

---

7 Ibid. p. 30.
8 Ibid. p. 44.

health. I even added more and more organic vegetables until I was consuming well over the four to six
requirement. I also added almond nut butter, for Dr.
Jensen spoke very highly about almonds and also indicated that they are the only alkaline nut. I liked
the butter very much and it was healthy for me.

In order to achieve a strong physical body, I was
determined to eat a very nutritious diet. Previously,
I had eliminated sugar, and I had never acquired a
taste for coffee. I also did not eat chocolate. My diet
had been quite healthy prior to this new information.
However, I had enjoyed a large amount of meat and
poultry. I was, by habit, a meat and potatoes eater.
This had to change. I reduced the amount of meat by
half and I attempted to eat the potato at a different
time of the day. More raw foods needed to be incorporated into my eating plan—salads helped to accomplish this. As I carefully altered my diet, I felt
better and even a sense of lightness in my body. I
needed to do everything to help my injured body.

My healing was being addressed from many directions. First, I had explored the mind and its power
to heal, enjoying a thorough hypnosis session every
week. I used my own tape and often updated it to fit
my new and evolving health issues. These enlightening sessions were also healing me emotionally as I allowed myself to be hopeful about my future. So this
directed the mental and emotional levels.

The energetic level was being healed by using the
NAET™ treatments. These opened the energy
meridians related to specific substances. They made
a very big difference. I also attended to my energy using the TAT™. This was the work of Tapas Fleming.
Her technique was instrumental in releasing the
blocks caused by traumas in my life. First, I worked
with the physical ones, such as minor surgeries, and
then I dealt with the emotional ones. The biggest one

was the exposure at the school. When I dealt with this, it required one month to process the release. This had been extremely traumatic and life-altering. However, when the processing was completed, I noticed an improvement in my health.

Further energetic blocks were being cleared by working with the "100 percent willing" technique. With all these efforts, I was trying to promote a clear and flowing energy system throughout my body.

Patricia and Robert also emphasized the energy of the body. They spoke of keeping me grounded and energetically strong. To help with being grounded, they told me to go outside and stand on the ground with my bare feet. This allows the energy to flow through the body into the earth. At first, I thought this seemed silly, but then I realized that I had always loved to walk barefoot outside. I always felt so calm and at one with nature. Perhaps there was more to it, now that I understood about energy. I became aware of my energy more and more. It is sad that in this country, our allopathic doctors aren't even aware that we need to protect our energy and make certain that it is free of blocks to ensure excellent health. Our well-being depends on an unimpeded energy flow throughout the body.

For the spiritual level, I continued to pray a rosary to the dear Divine Mother each day. There was a deep, close connection between us at this point. Whenever I asked a specific question and required assistance, it seemed that the answer came promptly. She seemed to be directing my way and I was honored to receive her guidance. With no idea what lay ahead of me, I stumbled along, with faith and hope in a new beginning.

Now, as a result of my recent studies with Trinity College of Natural Health, I was also attending to my physical body. I wanted to eat very nutritious food, work on building a healthy bloodstream, and reestablishing a strong, robust body. I was reminded of a quote by Hippocrates, "Let your food be your medicine and let your medicine be your food."[9]

So, at this point, I hoped I could reach deep within myself on many levels to bring about perfect glowing health. I realized that Environmental Illness is not a simple illness—easily healed with a few herbs or pills. It is a complex and serious problem, which involves many aspects of the body. I wanted to approach it from many angles to help bring my body back into balance. I needed to work on it from a *physical, emotional, mental, energetic,* and *spiritual level.*

As Barbara Ann Brennan, in her book *Hands of Light,* so nicely states, "In healing, there is no separation between body and mind, emotions and spirit— all need to be in balance to create a healthy human being."[10]

I was on my way. I only had to persevere until I reached my goal.

---

[9] Mark Pedersen, *Nutritional Herbology* (Warsaw, IN: Wensell W. Whitman Co. 1994), 1.

[10] Barbara Ann Brennan, *Hands of Light* (New York, NY: Bantam Books, 1988), 99.

PART V

*I look back at my work. I am relieved. It was hard,
but necessary. I extend a hand and encourage the
weary traveler to begin the healing journey across.*

Chapter 29

THE HEALER WITHIN

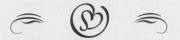

Gradually, that lonely autumn was nearing its conclusion as I continued studying and healing. My hesitancy to begin as a hypnotherapist was evident to Robert and Patricia. Gently, they kept hinting about my hypnosis ability. They were encouraging me to carry on with my life in a careful and safe way. They were right, but I was nervous about my future. I still had so far to go to heal myself. How would I be able to help others?

One day in early November, Eleanor, a very intelligent woman with whom I often spoke, phoned and asked me if I would be willing to do a session of hypnosis with her. She had been requesting this for some time, but I had avoided it. She had even hired another hypnotherapist to come to her home. This person had helped her relax but the therapist had no real knowledge of Environmental Illness. Eleanor was too ill to leave her home. I would have to go to her and I was a bit uncomfortable about this. She always talked about how her house made her sick. How would I be in her home? But, finally, I relented. We agreed on the next afternoon. When I arrived, she was holding a mask over her face and she was having a reaction to something. I went to a front bedroom, which was the only room she could use other than her own bedroom. She said she didn't know if she could relax—she was nervous. I didn't tell her, but I'm sure I was far more nervous than she was! This was my first official hypnosis session, and I wasn't sure what would result from it.

She rested on the bed. I had to stay in the corner of the room, as far away from her as possible, so I wouldn't cause her any problem with a scent I might have. There was no chair and so I stood in the corner. I began to go through a progressive relaxation. Eleanor closed her eyes. Then I realized that a strange feeling was coming over me. A surge of some kind of energy washed over my body. I became deeply relaxed and seemed to be lulled into an altered state as I spoke. Softly and naturally, my words flowed. She went under beautifully. She was a wonderful participant!

After the session, she peacefully opened her eyes and said that she felt very relaxed. I was so pleased that she could be so comfortable. The session had gone extremely well. I will always be very grateful to Eleanor for trusting me and letting me help her. It was the beginning of my hypnosis career.

The next week she asked me to come over again. I did not want to establish a career where I had to travel to each person's house. I still had Environmental Illness and I had to be very careful where I went. Also, it was a very long ride to her house, almost an hour. So, I made her a tape she could listen to at her leisure. Later I regretted this decision, for I could not monitor her and make sure that she came out of the trance properly. Also, I could not update the tape to meet her changing needs as her health evolved. Gradually, she also realized the problem involved and requested that I continue in person. We would have to figure out how to manage the situation.

One week after my session with Eleanor, another friend, Noreen, a member of the support group called me for a hypnosis session. She agreed to try to go to Dr. Sampson's office. We did the session there. This time, I could sit comfortably in a chair. The session went very smoothly. She was able to go into a nice relaxed state. Once again, as I began the session, I felt a strange feeling come over me. My voice even seemed to change. I wasn't sure what was happening. It seemed to happen as soon as I began to speak in my soft lilting voice. There was some kind of energy in the room and I did not understand where it was coming from.

So, I was now on my way, using hypnosis for people with Environmental Illness. The next person who called was yet another friend. However, she also could not leave her home. I talked with her on the phone and felt sorry that she was isolated in her home and not able to receive any treatment. That evening, David made a suggestion that changed my career. He thought that I should try to hypnotize her over the phone, since she had a speaker-phone. She could be safe and comfortable in her own home, and able to listen to my voice over the speaker. David's idea interested me. Perhaps this would be possible. At least this way I could make sure that she came out of the trance properly, by speaking with her after the session.

The next day, I called her. She seemed to like the idea. So, we experimented. It wasn't as good for me because I like to watch the person and make sure things are going well, but I was happy to compromise and help someone. It went well. This was a good suggestion of David's. We continued with this method for awhile. My friend's health improved and eventually she was able to go out and obtain the other treatments she needed. We continued the hypnosis on the phone, for it was a nice safe experience for her.

Now I had a new and wonderful tool to reach others who were extremely ill. We did not have to worry about the person being able to tolerate the office of Dr. Sampson. The person could rest at home and be helped. So, I started to assist others. Even people at long distances were now reachable.

I also kept working with Noreen at Dr. Sampson's office. She was responding beautifully to the suggestions. She preferred to work in person and so did I. She told me that an unfamiliar feeling came over her when she began the trance state. She felt that my voice held some kind of energy. This confirmed that something was indeed being experienced by both of us. Still, we weren't sure what it was.

After a few weeks of working with clients, I began to feel weak and dizzy. I didn't feel well. Patricia asked me if I had been taking care of my energy. I had no idea what she was talking about. She explained that, as a healer, I was channeling healing energy. Further, she explained that I needed to release the energy of my clients—energy that they are releasing during the session. She told me of a little prayer I could say to help me release and transmute the energy. After I learned to do this, I felt much better. Patricia informed me that now I was holding onto a higher vibration of energy. All of this seemed so foreign to me. I am so glad she educated me, for I needed to know how to handle all this new information.

This new role frightened me. I had never seen myself as a healer. I was even experiencing the changes going on within the person being hypnotized. I would have a certain sensation in my body and the person would relate the same feeling after the session. Once, the person even opened her eyes and told me she felt something strong happening within her body. I knew what she felt, for I, too, was experiencing it.

So much was happening and so much needed to be grasped that I decided to take a couple of weeks off. I needed to regroup and accept the new role. I also needed to let my energy become strong again. I had to slow down. I was only seeing a few people a week, but that was too much for me.

Winter was ending and I was becoming aware that my future was being formed—a future I needed to prepare for. Needing assistance of an even higher level, I placed a call to Dr. Leticia Oliver, Director of the Resource Center at the American Institute of Hypnotherapy. Once before, when I had spoken to her, I had felt a special connection. She was very knowledgeable and gifted about healing. When I told her of the latest developments, she understood. Very gently, she advised me to protect myself before the work with my clients by putting a vortex of light around my body. This light should move counter clockwise to repel negative energy and only allow in positive energy.

Also, I learned from another healer Eithel Lombardi, a wonderful and spiritual woman, that I should place a gold pyramid over my body to protect my energy.

I began to use these techniques, along with Patricia's prayer, at the end of the session. I noticed a great difference and my body seemed to be fine during the treatment. Very gradually, I commenced

again with my work and began to adapt to the idea
that I might have a little healing gift. However, one
day in early spring, an event occurred that altered
my life forever.

One lovely May day, I was sitting quietly in my
easy chair, holding my rosary beads and pondering
my new gift. Suddenly a light filled the room. I sat
back and looked up. A voice spoke gently and yet
firmly. The words were, "Touch them. It's your hands
that heal." I sat very still and waited. Nothing else
happened and the light returned to normal. What
was that? I had no idea.

The following day, again sitting quietly in my
chair, a smaller, less powerful voice repeated these
words. "Touch them. It's your hands that heal." This
time I was ready and I questioned. "Where do I touch
them?" In a moment the gentle voice answered, "We
show you."

"*We show you!*" What does that mean? I was baffled. Now I knew that I needed to talk to a person
about these recent transmissions. Nervously, I dialed
the number to speak with Dr. Oliver once again. Perhaps she might understand this message.

Sweetly, she responded to my inquiry, "Dear, you
are to be a healer with your hands. You must allow
divine guidance. Do not resist. They are going to prepare you to be a *healer.*"

There was that word again, "*healer!*"—now, *with
my hands!* I inquired, "But Dr. Oliver, WHO is speaking to me?" I felt silly asking this question.

Dr. Oliver spoke softly, "These are your guides." She
hesitated, "Some people call them your *ANGELS!*"

"ANGELS!" I was shaky. All my life I had seen de-
pictions of these gentle beings with graceful bodies
and wings, but I never imagined they would actually
contact ME!

I mustered the courage to go on with my line of questioning. I knew that Dr. Oliver was a busy person who was so graciously assisting me.

"Dr. Oliver, how will I know where to touch the person?"

She continued gently with words that stunned me, "Dear, they move your hands *for you.*"

No reply was possible for a moment.

She paused to allow me to process her news. Then she added, "It is very easy. Just hold your hands out in front of you and trust their guidance. They will be there for you."

This seemed too farfetched for me to grasp. However, I understood that something new and amazing was indeed occurring and I needed to be open—as open as I could be.

I thanked Dr. Oliver for her kindness. She encouraged me a bit more and then I replaced the receiver.

Tomorrow I would be seeing a client. Perhaps I could try and verify this information. Imagine! Angels moving my hands *for me!*

Prior to the session, I explained to Noreen about the new events that were unfolding. She was deeply moved. She somehow trusted me and encouraged me to try to use my hands to heal.

We began. I assisted her into a deep state of relaxation. This time I left out my "Angel of Healing" part, for I figured the angels would direct my hands to where she needed healing. I used a color visualization, end-result imagery, and some positive healing suggestions. At the culmination of the hypnosis session, I played very beautiful, spiritual music. I told her that she was divinely loved, and that the divine light of God was within her, protecting her and healing her. At that point, I stood up and moved closer to her body. Suddenly, a powerful feeling of healing energy came over me. My outstretched hands shook with this energy. They began to move into the prayer position. It was real! The angels were working. I began to pray for my client, but suddenly, my hands were moved apart and extended over her body to work on healing. They drifted over her and centered on certain areas. I watched in amazement! My hands continued to shake with this divine energy and a deep feeling of divine love filled my essence. After working for only a few moments, the angels signaled their completion by returning my hands to the prayer position. I had never experienced anything like this before! This day would change the rest of my life. There would be no more doubts!

When my client returned to a waking state, she asked me what had just happened to her. I asked her what she had felt. She explained that she had been placed in a gold pyramid of light and then she saw angels all around her! We shared our tears of astonishment and felt deeply blessed to share this divine healing.

I am extremely pleased and honored that the Blessed Mother has bestowed this gift upon me. I am very new at healing and I don't know what the future holds. I only know that I am here for a purpose and I will do my best to give whatever I can.

After this event, I recalled a strange experience from the past. A few years before, I had been taking a walk through the forest with my husband. A woman was strolling near us and began to converse with us. She was very educated and knowledgeable about health. She looked at me intently and asked if I were a healer. I laughed and replied that I was a teacher. She was very thoughtful. She shook her head. She said that she was sure that I was a healer. Still, I insisted that I was a teacher and that I had no intention of being a healer. She would not relent. Finally, as we parted, she said, "You may not be a healer now, but you will be!"

These words came back to me. Could she have known something that I did not? Only time will tell and I will just await the answers.

Chapter 30

WHAT'S GOING TO HAPPEN TO ME?

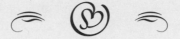

"**W**hat's going to happen to me?" These are the words I find myself uttering when I look out the window and wonder about my future. I have no idea what will happen to me. I am now a different person than I was four and a half years ago. I am not even sure in what ways I have changed, but I know I have changed. I have had to in order to survive. One major way I have changed is that I don't try to make life the way I want it to be. I don't force issues. I let the "Divine plan" take its route. I just do my best with what I have and I wait to see what I need to do next. There is so much to the world that I cannot control and that I do not comprehend. I have learned so much and I have so much more to learn.

I wish I could close this book and say about my injury, "All set, fini, easy come easy go, or piece of cake." I wish I could wipe my hands of the illness and say I had made history of it, but I cannot. Healing from Environmental Illness is a complicated and

long journey. I am still on this healing journey. At
least I can say that I am over the horrible part of the
injury, when I was close to death. Just last month,
one of my clients confided in me that when she used
to call me and speak with me, she used to hang up
and pray to God. She used to say, "Please God, don't
let me get as sick as Lorri." She told me this now because she is amazed at how I have improved. She
now strives to be well like I am and so she does hypnosis with me to encourage her subconscious to direct her healing. Another friend told me that when
she used to call each day, she wondered if I would be
still alive. I was that ill!

So, now I am able to live in my home and wear cotton clothes. I can be nice and warm after a shower,
and I can sit comfortably in my favorite easy chair.
My world is opening up and my body is stronger. I am
able to read books easily without the need for my
glass table. I can type on my computer for a much
longer time than fifteen minutes! I can watch television and even have the television in the same room
with me! I can talk on a regular phone for as long as
I wish. Music is an important part of my life again
and I can play my piano. I have assembled a lovely,
colorful wardrobe of cotton clothes and have many
pretty outfits to wear. Even the light is easier for me
now. I am able to go in my car at any time with only
one pair of sunglasses. I am almost able to take a
walk outside in the light. This will come. Also, just
this week I strolled through a department store with
absolutely no difficulty. So much is better!

I guess that sometimes it is a strange blessing to
lose the simple things in life. So many people seem to
need to have new cars, jewelry, and designer clothes
to feel happy in life. When they dress hastily in the
morning and take a casual shower, they may not re-

alize that in those acts alone, they have been given great gifts. I totally enjoy the action of putting on my nice clean clothes and a different outfit from the day before. I thank God each time I can do this. I delight in the warmth of a towel around my body after a shower. This is so wonderful to be able to do again. If only others could see how lucky they are in having the simple gifts that are so special. I hope to always be grateful for these moments.

What I would like to impart with this book is hope for those of you who are in the midst of this devastating illness. For you who have lost belief in yourself and your future, it is important to know that there are new and excellent ways to open the energy meridians of the body and to clear the allergies. There are ways to reach deep into the subconscious and help usher the body out of the intense illness. There are answers happening all the time, as more and more awareness is dawning. *Be open to what is around you and allow the healing process to begin.*

I think the most important thing to do is to remove the limitations from our lives. I realize that we cannot remove the allergies and sensitivities easily, but I am speaking of the mental limitations. As Norman Vincent Peale once said:

> A truly tragic fact that we must face is that many people settle for—and actually practice—their limitations. They practice them so constantly and for so long a time that the limitations become habits. A person comes to be frozen into his limitations much like a polar ship frozen into the Arctic Ocean, so that it cannot move.[1]

---

[1] Norman Vincent Peale, *How to Handle Tough Times* (Pawling, NY: Peale Center for Christian Living, 1990), 13.

We cannot allow the present mind set toward Environmental Illness of "no way out" to prevail. The body can heal and the spirit can become enriched once again. It takes time and effort. Most of all it takes courage—more than anyone can imagine. To persevere when there are no clear answers and no messages of hope is so challenging, but it must be done! Today, upon the completion of this book, I pray I have brought you some degree of hope. There is a way out and there can be a wonderful future ahead for you!

Begin the way by opening your mind and seeking answers. You can become a useful and respected member of the community once again. You can begin by planning for a life that may be possible in the future. I needed to plan and reach for some kind of goal so that I could feel there was a reason to heal and move forward. Because I wasn't sure to what degree I could recover, I didn't know if I could return to teach in a classroom with thirty teenagers all wearing perfume and after-shave lotion. (Also, each girl often prided herself with perfect hairstyles held in place with pounds of hairspray.) This situation might not be easy for me in my future, so I have had to tailor my plans to meet my new requirements.

I planned for the time when I could venture out again into the world! I would need to work in a private practice and with one client at a time. This way I could request that the person not wear fragrances. Also, I would want to monitor my work environment, so that renovations were not being carried on while I was trying to work. All this needed to be considered.

This is one of the reasons I studied hypnosis, along with the need to heal my mind. I hoped that maybe someday I could work in the field of hypnosis. And now, even though I may only see a few people a week and don't earn enough to pay for one week's grocery bill, I feel like I am worthwhile. I feel like I am a human being who matters again.

We each can seek to find a new career or purpose because it is so vital to feel needed and useful. Even if a person cannot return to his prior career, perhaps a new endeavor can be rewarding and help to rebuild a broken self-esteem.

I send this message at a time when I, too, am still working on my healing journey. It would be easy to rebuild my life if I had no limitations and were completely well, but it is more important for me to rebuild it now so that I can feel that my life is worth saving and living. I hope I can help others with EI to go on and find their bright futures. Perhaps we can play a role as the wounded healers. By learning from our own illness, we can give so much empathy and kindness to others who are in the midst of this devastating and debilitating problem.

Society's Role

For others in our society who are living with people with EI, I would ask you to give them love and respect. Even if you cannot understand this illness, believe in your loved one. If you think it is hard to understand, believe me it is even harder for the person with EI to comprehend. There is much that is not clear about this illness. One thing is certain: EI is indeed **REAL** and **VERY SERIOUS!** The medical community needs to address it and consider it of the highest priority! Too many people are suffering without the support of the traditional medical doctors! Sufficient research is necessary to explain, heal, and prevent this extremely serious condition.

We all need to examine our environments and our surroundings. This includes not only the chemicals and substances we breathe and handle, but also the people with whom we associate and the attitudes we are handling. If our coworkers are constantly negative and destructive, we, too, will feel this force in our energy system.

We also need to breathe clean fresh air as much as possible!

When a person becomes ill from a poor and unhealthy environment, believe in that person. Help the individual recover and respect his/her efforts to do so. Please don't put a person with EI in a closet to be forgotten.

We are still important, so please keep us involved with the world. Talk to us and include us in events. Invite us, even if we may not be able to attend. It requires special effort, but please help us remain part of your lives.

More importantly, encourage a person with EI to get well. Give the person hope and belief in the power to heal. Look into new and interesting ways to heal the body and mind. Give a positive outlook and say positive comments. If the person is unable to read books or use a computer, research for him/her. Seek out answers and support the healing process.

One very small but important difference you can make is simply to call! Call and care! Take the extra few moments out of your busy day to remember a person who is confined and sad. This can brighten a day more than you can ever imagine! Environmental Illness can be a very lonely time and connections are difficult to maintain. Be there and help the person know he/she is still valuable and loved!

Someday, perhaps there will be clear answers, so that when a person is injured by chemical fumes or other substances in the environment, an easy solution will be known. I dream of this day. But, for now, a deep and emotional healing journey is called for.

Most of All . . .

Take the first step into the healing journey. At the beginning, the process is slow and laborious. Later, as you heal, it moves faster and you feel increasingly better. Your life will open up and your activities will expand.

When I first became ill, many people said that once you get Environmental Illness, you are never the same. I used to be very disheartened when I heard this. I wanted to return to the same person I was before the injury, but now I know I could never go back. This is truly a transformational illness. There is so much to learn and understand. The experience can be so enriching. You will develop an understanding of yourself, your needs, and the world around you. Perhaps you will understand the forces that made you ill and you can play a role in changing the negative energies that surround you. Instead of tolerating them, you can transform them. Perhaps you can even add enrichment to the lives of others from your wonderful discoveries.

Perhaps it would be nicer to hope that you will not be the same. You will be, in many ways, *better.*

The pieces were beginning to fit together and I was reclaiming my life! Yet there remained one message repeating in my mind from my friendly neighbor Ping. Her words, "Lorri, don't die!" had echoed in my ears since they were delivered.

Chapter 31

HELLO . . . PING . . .

*T*here was one more thing I had to do to finish business. My healing journey was well under way and I was much stronger. Daily survival was no longer a struggle. I owed Ping a phone call. Her powerful telephone message, two years earlier, had sustained me throughout my healing adventure.

I called her. We chatted for a few minutes. She was delighted to hear from me. Before we used to talk while we worked on our gardens and our flowers, but since my injury, I had not been able to go outside. She hadn't seen me in over three years.

After we talked for awhile, it was time to hang up. This time, it was I who ended the conversation. I said, "Ping, I made it. I didn't die!"

APPENDIX

Included here are the names, addresses, and phone numbers of some of the practitioners I have mentioned. Also listed are schools, and items of interest covered in my book

American Institute of Hypnotherapy
16842 Von Karman Avenue, Suite 475
Irvine, CA 92714
Phone: 1–800–872–9996

"Believe, Just Believe" (cassette)
See in back of book
Diveena Publications
P.O. Box 413
Chelmsford, MA 01824

Tapas Fleming
TAT™ International
P.O. Box 7000–379
Redondo, CA 90277
Phone: 1–877–828–4685
www.tat-intl.com

Dr. Devi Nambudripad
6714 Beach Blvd.
Buena Park, CA 90621
Phone: 1–714–523–8900

Network Chiropractic
(Now termed, Network Spinal Analysis)
Donald Epstein
444 North Main St.
Longmont, CO 80501

Dr. Robert Sampson and Patricia Hughes
P.O. Box 940
Londonderry, NH 03053-0940
Phone: 1–603–537–1200

Trinity School of Natural Health
810 S. Buffalo St.
Warsaw, IN 46580–4101
Phone: 1–800–428–0408

Books dealing with the symptoms and resolutions of problems resulting from *candida albicans* (yeast):

The Yeast Connection and the Woman
William G. Crook, M.D.
Professional Books, Inc.
Box 3246
Jackson, Tennessee 38303

Back to Health
Dennis W. Remington, M.D.
Barbara W. Higa, R.D.
Vitality House, International, Inc.
1675 North Freedom, Blvd. #11–C
Provo, Utah 84604
Phone: 1–800–637–0708

Included here are the names of companies that carry products for the environmentally aware and the chemically sensitive person.

Cosmetics—fragrance-free

Annemarie Borlind
P.O. Box 130
New London, NH 03257
Phone: 1–800–447–7024

Ecco Bella Botanicals
1133 Rt. 23
Wayne, NJ 07470

Cotton Clothing

Lands' End,
1 Lands' End Lane
Dodgeville, WI 53595
Phone: 1–800–356–4444

Reflections Organic
P.O. Box 1999
North Bend, WA 98045
Phone: 1–800–852–9273
(100% organic cotton)

Natural Products for the Home

Harmony (Seventh Generation)
360 Interlocken Boulevard, Suite 300
Broomfield, CO 80021
Phone: 1–800–869–3446
(Natural products for the home)

Intertherm electric heaters now sold by:
Cadet Manufacturing Co.
P.O. Box 1675
Vancouver, WA 98668-1675
Phone: 1–360–693–2505

Janice Corp.
198 Route 46
Budd Lake, NJ 07828
Phone: 1–800 JANICES
(Natural bedding, clothing, and personal care
   products)

The Living Source
P.B. Box 20155
Waco, Texas 76702
Phone: 1–254–776–4878
(Personal care, books, air filters, etc.)

N.E.E.D.S.
527 Charles Avenue, 12–A
Syracuse, NY 13209
Phone: 1–800–634–1380
(Personal care, books, air filters, etc.)

Pacific International Group, Inc.
Phone: 1–800–797–7007
(Laundry disks)

Soaps—fragrance-free

Coastline Products
P.O. Box 6397
Santa Ana, CA 92706
Phone: 1–800–554–4112
(Simple soap and other fragrance-free cleaning
   products)

Vitamins and Herbs

The Vitamin Shoppe
Phone: 1–800–223–1216
(reduced prices on vitamins, herbs, and personal care
products)

BIBLIOGRAPHY

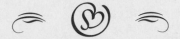

Brennan, Barbara Ann. *Hands of Light*. New York, NY: Bantam Books, 1988.

Burton Goldberg Group. *Alternative Medicine*. Fife, WA: Future Medicine Publishing, Inc., 1994.

Chopra, Deepak, M.D. *Quantum Healing: Exploring The Frontiers of Mind/Body Medicine*. New York, NY: Bantam Books, 1989.

Cousins, Norman. *Anatomy of an Illness*. New York, NY: Bantam Books, 1981.

Dewe, Bruce A., M.D. and Joan R. Dewe, MA. *Professional Kinesiology Practice II: Advanced Specialised Kinesiology Methods*. Auckland, New Zealand: Professional Health Publications, 1997. PKP Certification Programme™: www.icpkp.com

Fleming, Tapas, L.Ac. *Reduce Traumatic Stress in Minutes*. Torrance, CA: TAT™ Workbook, 1996.

Hilgard, Ernest R. and Josephine R. Hillgard. *Hypnosis in the Relief of Pain*. New York, NY: Brunner/Mazel, 1994.

Ivker, Robert, M.D. *Sinus Survival.* Los Angeles, CA: Jeremy P. Tarcher, Inc., 1992.

Jensen, Bernard, Ph.D. *The Chemistry of Man.* Escondido, CA: Bernard Jensen International, 1983.

Korn, Errol R. and Karen Johnson. *Visualization: The Uses of Imagery in the Health Professions.* Homewood, IL: Dow Jones-Irwin, 1983.

Krasner, A. M., Ph.D. *The Wizard Within.* Santa Anna, CA: American Board of Hypnotherapy Press, 1991.

Lawson, Lynn. *Staying Well in a Toxic World.* Chicago, IL: The Noble Press, Inc. 1993.

Miller, Emmett E. *Deep Healing: The Essence of Mind/Body Medicine.* Carlsbad, CA: Hay House, Inc., 1997.

Morter, M. Ted Jr., D.C. *Your Health . . . Your Choice.* Hollywood, FL: Lifetime Books, Inc., 1995.

Nambudripad, Devi, S., D.C., L.Ac., R.N., Ph.D. *Say Goodbye to Illness.* Buena Park, CA: Delta Publishing Co., 1993.

Peale, Norman Vincent. *How to Handle Tough Times.* Pawling, NY: Peale Center for Christian Living, 1990.

Pedersen, Mark. *Nutritional Herbology.* Warsaw, IN: Wendell W. Whitman Co., 1994.

Robbins, Anthony. *Unlimited Power.* New York, NY: Ballantine Books, 1987.

Rochlitz, Steven Prof. *Allergies and Candida: with the Physicist's Rapid Solution.* Mahopac, NY: Human Ecology Balancing Sciences, Inc., 1995.

Rosen, Sidney. *My Voice Will Go with You: The Teaching Tales of Milton H. Erickson.* New York, NY: W. W. Norton & Company, 1991.

Sampson, Robert, M.D. and Patricia Hughes, B.S.N. *Breaking Out of Environmental Illness.* Santa Fe, NM: Bear & Company, 1997.

Simonton, O. Carl, M.D. and Stephanie Matthews Simonton. *Getting Well Again.* New York, NY: Bantam Books, 1992.

GLOSSARY

acupressure: the massaging of points along the energy meridians

acupuncture: the use of needles placed in energy meridians to open the pathways

ADR, Accidental Disability Retirement: a pension granted by the state to workers who have paid into the teachers retirement system.

allergen: a substance that provokes allergic reactions

allergies: energy blockages due to contact with adverse energies

alternative medicine: selection of treatments that differ from those of traditional allopathic medical doctors

angels: divine beings of light

baquet: tub

biofeedback: a system to monitor the internal processes of the body in order to correct them

brain fog: difficulty thinking clearly as a result of exposure to an allergenic substance

candida: a yeast that normally grows in the intestinal tract. (During times of health impairment these yeasts can overgrow causing health problems.)

chakra: an energy center in the body

conscious mind: the logical, analytical mind— represents alert awareness

Division of Occupational Hygiene: an agency that monitors the air quality in buildings

energy blockage: an interference in the electrical flow in or around the body

energy meridian: a pathway of electrical impulse in the body

EPD, Enzyme Potentiated Desensitization: an injection of minute levels of many allergens to stimulate immune building response to them

environmental medicine: the study and treatment of symptoms resulting from environmental exposures

foot reflexology: the massaging of acupressure points on the sides and bottom of the foot to bring about health improvement

fresh air: air that is clear of high levels of allergens (including chemicals)

gate point: a specific location along the energy meridian

hypersensitivity: allergies resulting in obvious physical reactions, for example, sneezing, coughing, or wheezing

hypnosis: derived from the Greek word, *hypnos,* meaning sleep. A deeply relaxed state wherein the subconscious mind can be easily accessed.

hyposensitivity: hidden allergies resulting in poor general health

iridology: the study of the body's health by examining the patterns in the iris of the eye

kinesiology: muscle-testing

laundry discs: small plastic shells with tiny ceramic balls inside, altering the ionic composition of water so that dirt is pulled off clothes

MACI, Massachusetts Association for the Chemically Injured: a support group

MCS/EI, Multiple Chemical sensitivity/Environmental Illness: a serious health condition evidenced by reactions to chemicals at exposure levels considered to be extremely low for the general population

meningeal tension: stress found in the sheath surrounding the spinal chord

MSDS sheets: Material Safety Data Sheets prepared by the manufacturer of chemicals that explain the proper usage and possible side effects of the product

muscle testing: applying pressure to a particular muscle to determine its strength or weakness in order to obtain information from the body

NAET, Nambudripad Allergy Elimination Technique: an allergy clearing method using the stimulation of acupressure points

naturopathy: a natural approach to enhance the immune system. Often the use of herbs and vitamins is included.

Network Chiropractic: a spinal adjustment method developed from a combination of chiropractic techniques, created by Donald Epstein

obsolete programming: inappropriate response from a program set into action during a past event

OSHA: Occupation Safety and Health Agency

outgas: the release of fumes into the air

photophobia: sensitivity to light

reading box: a glass box with metal trim, constructed to fit over a book

reframing: viewing a problem from a new perspective

rishis: ancient men of wisdom from India

sensory nerve fiber: a nerve leading from the spinal chord

spreading: the addition of more and more allergies

subconscious mind: the emotional mind, accessible during a relaxed state

trauma: an event in life that results in an energy blockage

Veda: ancient books of wisdom from India

vial: a tiny glass container

workers compensation: a state-based insurance program directed by the Division of Industrial Accidents to pay workers a portion of their salaries in case of injury while working

INDEX

Also Available from

Diveena ♡ Publications

Believe, Just Believe

A cassette of Christian songs performed by
Lorri Smith

Experience the healing energy of Lorri's inspired songs!

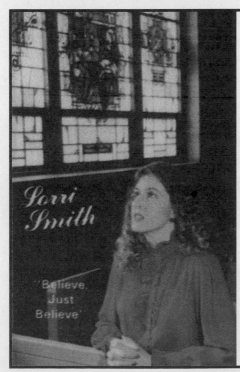

Side A
1. **Believe, Just Believe*
2. *He*
3. *Romans Eight*
4. *How Great Thou Art*

Side B
1. *Gentle Shepherd*
2. **When I Need God*
3. *Let There Be Peace on Earth*
4. ***I Lift My Eyes to the Lord*
5. *I Believe*

*Lyrics and music by
Lorri Smith

**Lyrics: Psalm 121, music by
Lorri Smith

Gentle Shepherd written by
Fr. McDonough

When I Need God awarded *Billboard Magazine's*
Certificate of Achievement, 1991.

ORDER FORM

Heal Environmental Illness and Reclaim Your Life!

Please send _____ books to :
              (quantity)

Name: _____

Address: _____

City: _____

State: _____   Zip: _____

Telephone: (_____) _____

Believe, Just Believe

Please send _____ tapes to :
              (quantity)

Name: _____

Address: _____

City: _____

State: _____   Zip: _____

Telephone: (_____) _____

Price per book:
$14.95 plus $3.00 shipping and handling

Price per cassette:
$10.00 plus $2.00 shipping and handling

Sales Tax:
Please add 5.0% for items shipped to Massachusetts.

Special Offer:
Orders over $20.00—free shipping and handling!

Please send check or money order to:

> Diveena Publications
> P. O. Box 413
> Chelmsford, MA 01824

I have enclosed a check in the amount of _____

NOTES

NOTES